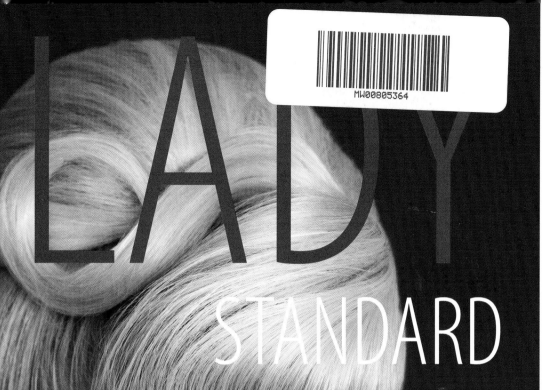

MILADY

STANDARD

Timothy C. Johnson

UPDOS

CENGAGE
Learning®

Australia • Brazil • Japan • Korea • Mexico • Singapore • Spain • United Kingdom • United States

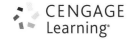

Milady Standard Updos
Timothy C. Johnson

Executive Director, Milady: Sandra Bruce

Product Director: Corina Santoro

Product Manager: Philip I. Mandl

Product Team Manager: Julie Shepperly

Senior Content Developer: Jessica Mahoney

Associate Content Developer: Sarah Prediletto

Director, Marketing & Training: Gerard McAvey

Community Manager: Matthew McGuire

Senior Production Director: Wendy Troeger

Production Manager: Sherondra Thedford

Senior Content Project Manager: Stacey Lamodi

Senior Art Director: Benj Gleeksman

Cover image(s): Copyright © 2015 Milady,
a part of Cengage Learning®. Photography
by Timothy C. Johnson.

For product information and technology assistance, contact us at
Cengage Learning Customer & Sales Support, 1-800-354-9706

For permission to use material from this text or product,
submit all requests online at **www.cengage.com/permissions.**
Further permissions questions can be e-mailed to
permissionrequest@cengage.com

Library of Congress Control Number: 2013950589

ISBN-13: 978-1-2854-4449-9

Cengage Learning
5 Maxwell Drive
Clifton Park, NY 12065-2919
USA

Cengage Learning is a leading provider of customized learning solutions with office locations around the globe, including Singapore, the United Kingdom, Australia, Mexico, Brazil, and Japan. Locate your local office at:
international.cengage.com/region

Cengage Learning products are represented in Canada by Nelson Education, Ltd.

For your lifelong learning solutions, visit **milady.cengage.com**

Purchase any of our products at your local college store or at our preferred online store **www.cengagebrain.com**

Visit our corporate website at **cengage.com**.

Notice to the Reader

Publisher does not warrant or guarantee any of the products described herein or perform any independent analysis in connection with any of the product information contained herein. Publisher does not assume, and expressly disclaims, any obligation to obtain and include information other than that provided to it by the manufacturer. The reader is expressly warned to consider and adopt all safety precautions that might be indicated by the activities described herein and to avoid all potential hazards. By following the instructions contained herein, the reader willingly assumes all risks in connection with such instructions. The publisher makes no representations or warranties of any kind, including but not limited to, the warranties of fitness for particular purpose or merchantability, nor are any such representations implied with respect to the material set forth herein, and the publisher takes no responsibility with respect to such material. The publisher shall not be liable for any special, consequential, or exemplary damages resulting, in whole or part, from the readers' use of, or reliance upon, this material.

Printed in the United States of America
1 2 3 4 5 6 7 18 17 16 15 14

CONTENTS

ABOUT THE AUTHOR

Timothy C. Johnson began his career at Vidal Sassoon in Chicago. He later moved to Milan, Italy, where he started his career in fashion, styling hair for photo shoots, runway shows, and commercials. His work has appeared in *Vogue, Vanity Fair, Glamour, Marie Claire, O: The Oprah Magazine*, and more. Assignments have taken him all over the world. His first book, *Red Carpet Hair: Beautiful Hairstyles for Special Occasions,* was published in 2011. Timothy currently resides in New York City.

ACKNOWLEDGMENTS

Thank you God for your constant blessings.

Thank you Mom and Dad, Elmira Smith, and Arthur Johnson, for your love and support.

Thank you to Philip Mandl and Martine Edwards. Jessica Mahoney, it was a pleasure to work with you and thank you for your efficiency!

A special thanks goes to Aliesh Pierce and Anastacia Berzat.

Thank you to all the assistants who helped me with this project: Imani Razat, Malwina Augustyn, Elizabeth Rim, Shawn Alexandra Ilardi-Lony, Saidia Neblett, and Deirdre Thompson.

To all the beautiful models, thank you, thank you, thank you, for your time and patience. I could not have done it without you: Paige Grimard, Stefanie Raben, Rennishol John, Malwina Augustyn, Elizabeth Rim, Whitney Buck, Brigid Turner, and Kadeja Wexler.

Reviewers

The author and publisher wish to acknowledge the following professionals for their support in the development of the manuscript by providing recommendations to help shape the final product.

Crystal A. Rivenbark, Hair Architecture, LLC, Midlothian, VA
Dawn Medina, Medina Hair Design, Fort Wayne, IN
Heather Murdoch, Guru Salon and Spa, Falmouth, ME
Janet Prediletto, Janet Prediletto Professional Aesthetics LTD,
    Saratoga Springs, NY
Linda Garcia, Independent Stylist, Rio Rancho, NM
Olivia Hill, The Hair Junkies Salon Studio, Allen, TX
Sandy LeClear, Trend Setters, Fort Wayne, IN
Tyler Fedigan, Saratoga Springs Massage Therapy, LLC, Corinth, NY

INTRODUCTION

The red carpet has a tremendous influence on our cultural fascination with great hairstyles. From Oscar night to the Golden Globes, clients request the hairstyles worn by celebrities at red-carpet events, styles often inspired by those of old Hollywood. Many of these hairstyles are classic updos that were worn by actresses and musicians such as Audrey Hepburn, Grace Kelly, Elizabeth Taylor, Diana Ross, Julia Roberts, and the list goes on. Every hairstylist should pay close attention to the red carpet to predict the latest trends. The updo is a lucrative service for the stylist and the salon, so don't underestimate its earning power!

The main concept behind *Milady Standard Updos* is to demonstrate the different techniques for putting the hair up. The updos demonstrated are based on classic hairstyles inspired by the red carpet. Learning the classics is imperative to mastering updos. Some fashion-forward hairstyles are also featured. A great foundation gives you the freedom to create these and many other styles.

Tools introduces all of the supplies that you will need to create. Having the proper combs, brushes, fasteners, and products in your arsenal will enable you to achieve the best results for any updo, no matter the client's hair length or texture.

As discussed in the *Preparation* section, five steps are critical to getting your updo started. First, consult with the client and decide what hairstyle you are going to do. Second, drape the client by adding a neck strip, or thin towel and cape. Third, shampoo and condition the hair. We worked with clean hair for all of the styles shown in the book. The fourth step is blowdrying. Sometimes rollers and pin curls are added during or after blowdrying. Wet sets are another option for the fourth step. The fifth step is adding or subtracting texture, which means to curl or flat iron the hair, and this step is optional.

There are eight categories of updos in this book: Half Up, Ponytail, Chignon, Bun on Top, French Twist, Faux Bob, Up in Pieces, and Tousled Up. Three to four updos are demonstrated in each category, showing variations on each theme. Women of different ethnicities and hair textures are featured throughout the book to give insight on working with the various hair textures.

You may ask why ponytails and half-up hairstyles are included in an updo book. They are included because some clients are not comfortable with all of their hair up. You get the best of both worlds with these styles—the client gets to have some hair down while the rest of the hair is securely in place.

Milady Standard Updos will give students and hairstylists the necessary tools to become skilled at updos. This book is filled with techniques and ideas for constructing any updo. Being proficient at updos and styling hair for special occasions gives you an advantage over the competition and improves your earning potential. The intent of *Milady Standard Updos* is to inspire creativity, and the opportunity for stylists to express their artistic abilities.

TOOLS

The following tools are needed for preparing and creating an updo. You should be familiar with most of these items already. Be sure to add these tools to your kit if you are missing any because they will be helpful for constructing updos.

Combs

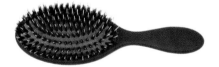

Styling comb with lift

The styling comb with lift creates a smooth surface and the lift elevates the hair.

Tail comb

The tail comb creates a smooth surface and the tail end is used to section and arrange the hair.

Teasing comb

The teasing comb is used to make a cushion at the base of the hair for added volume.

Wide-tooth comb

The wide-tooth comb is essential for detangling and combing out wet hair.

Brushes

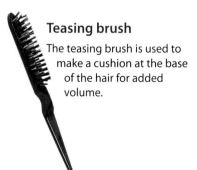

Cushion brush

The cushion brush or nylon-bristle brush is used for smoothing out the top layer of teased hair, styling, and detangling.

Teasing brush

The teasing brush is used to make a cushion at the base of the hair for added volume.

Paddle brush

The paddle brush is used to detangle hair when wet and is also used as blowdry brush. Paddle brushes have large, flat bases and are well suited for mid-length to longer-length hair. Some have ball-tipped nylon pins and staggered pin patterns that help keep the hair from snagging.

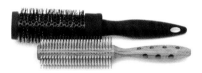

Round brush

The round brush is used to smooth and add body to the hair.

Vent brush

The vent brush is used to add lift to the roots of the hair, and it is also used to dry and style hair.

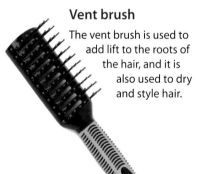

Heat Styling

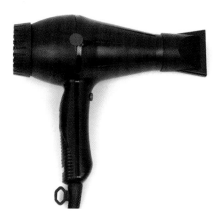

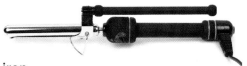

Curling iron

The curling iron is a heat styling tool that curls and smoothes the hair.

Blowdryer

A blowdryer is an electrical appliance designed for drying and styling hair.

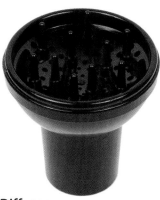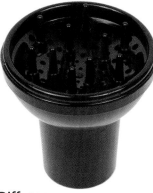

Flat iron

The flat iron is a heat styling tool that straightens and smoothes the hair.

Diffuser

A diffuser is an attachment added to the blowdryer to dry curly hair. The diffuser causes the air to flow more softly, and helps to accentuate or keep textural definition.

Fillers

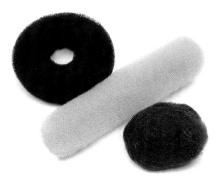

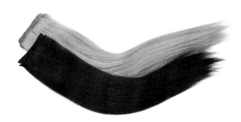

Wefts

Wefts are long strips of human or artificial hair with a threaded edge. A weft of hair adds extra length and fullness to the hair.

Fillers

Fillers, which are available in a variety of shapes and sizes, add fullness and form to an updo.

Fasteners

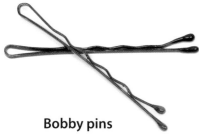

Bobby pins

Bobby pins are used to hold the hair in place. Bobby pins are available in a variety of colors to closely resemble a client's hair color.

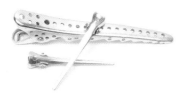

Clips

Clips are used to temporarily hold hair and rollers in place. Various sizes are available; large clips are ideal for sectioning. They are usually made of metal or plastic and have long prongs to hold wet or dry sections of hair in place.

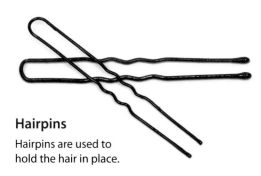

Hairpins

Hairpins are used to hold the hair in place.

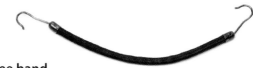

Bungee band

A bungee band is a band with two hooks at the end used to hold ponytails in place.

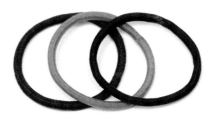

Elastic bands

Elastic bands are used to hold ponytails in place.

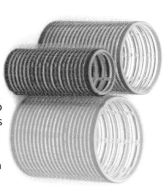

Rollers

Rollers are used to add body to the hair. Note that the author chose to use Velcro rollers for this title. Some state boards do not allow Velcro rollers because they can be difficult to clean and disinfect. Be sure to check with your state board before selecting rollers.

Additional Supplies

- **Conditioner**
- **Capes**
- **Foam or mousse**

- **Gel (straightening gel and liquid gel)**
- **Hairspray (finishing or texture spray)**
- **Neck strips**

- **Pomade (wax)**
- **Shampoo (wet and dry)**
- **Towels**

PREPARATION

After consulting with a client and choosing the updo, the preparation of the hair is the foundation for creating an updo. The hair should first be shampooed and conditioned, and the appropriate styling product should be added. The texture of the hair helps determine the look of an updo. Sometimes the hair goes from curly to straight or from straight to curly in an updo—whichever texture is needed, make sure to leave some body in the hair. When the client's hair has the appropriate body and the proper product(s) applied, you will have better control over the hair; it also makes teasing easier. Prepare the hair properly and it will help form the updo. Blowdrying, rollers, pin curls, and curling irons are used to prepare the hair for an updo.

Blowdrying

When blowdrying the hair for an updo, in most cases you want to add fullness and body to make the construction of the updo easier. First apply the proper styling product(s) to the hair. Then begin blowdrying the hair to take some of the moisture out, using your hands to move the hair from side to side while drying. Sometimes a vent brush is used to lift the roots, depending on the texture of the hair. Use large clips to keep the damp hair out of the way. Then, taking 2-inch sections, dry the hair with a round brush or flat brush, starting from the front or back of the head. Make sure to dry the root area first for good root lift. Rollers and pin curls can be added for maximum root lift and to give fullness to the hair, either during or after the blowdry. Curling irons and flat irons are used after blowdrying to enhance curls or smooth the hair.

Rollers

Rollers are a great way to add fullness and body to the hair. Add rollers as you dry each section for maximum root lift and fullness. Start with the front. If the style has a side part, roll the first roller to the side; if not, roll it back. After all rollers have been added, apply a light hair spray and then let the hair cool for 1 to 5 minutes. After the hair cools, brush the hair with a vent or nylon-bristle brush to eliminate the parts made by the roller sections.

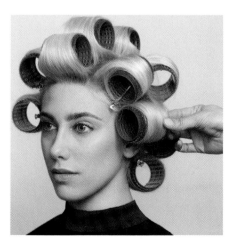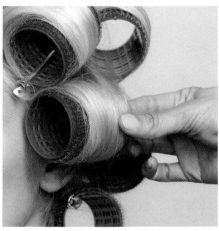

Pin Curls

Pin curling is another way of creating maximum root lift and fullness. Pin curls give a slightly tighter curl and add more texture than rollers. As each section is dried, wrap the section around one or two fingers and clip it at the roots to secure, making sure the ends are tucked inside the curl. If the style has a side part, pin the curl to the side; if not, pin the curl back. After the pin curls are finished, add a light hair spray and allow the hair to cool for 1 to 5 minutes. Finger through the pin curls or brush through them with a nylon-bristle brush.

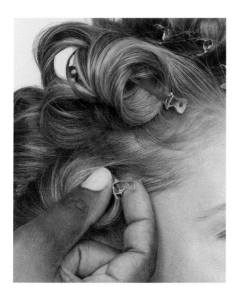 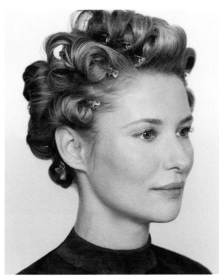

Curling Irons

The curling iron is used for tighter curls or to smooth the hair after blowdrying. Use a light hair spray on each curl for extended hold. After cooling for 1 to 5 minutes, the curls should be fingered through or brushed through with a nylon-bristle brush depending on the hairstyle.

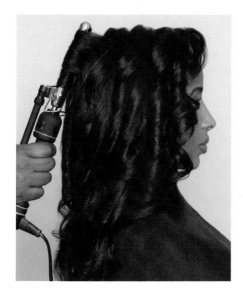 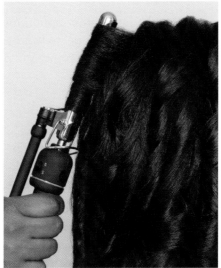

Straightening Hair

Going from curly to straight requires a smoothing product, brush, and blow-dryer. Make sure to leave some body in the hair. If the hairstyle doesn't require curl or lots of volume, the hair can be blown out with body and not be put into rollers or pin curls. Sometimes no body is needed at all; it really depends on the hairstyle. Flat irons can also be used to smooth the hair for sleeker hairstyles.

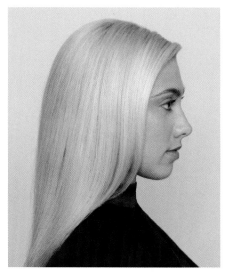 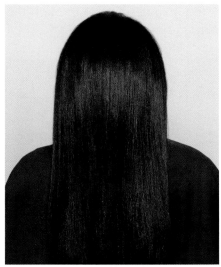

Other Options for Preparation

- Wet sets are used to straighten, add body, or add curl to naturally curly and chemically relaxed hair.
- Curly hair can also be dried with a diffuser on the end of the blowdryer so that it dries naturally without frizz.
- Heat rollers are another tool that can be used after blowdrying to add body.
- For extremely tight ponytails, blowdry the hair straight without adding body.
- Molding is another option for sleek ponytails. When molding, apply a setting lotion or gel to wet hair. Comb the hair in the desired direction using a fine tooth comb, and place the client under a hooded dryer.

Teasing

Teasing increases the hair's volume and helps it to stay in place. It also creates a cushion on which to latch bobby pins and hairpins. It can be done only near the scalp or at the scalp and the ends. Sometimes just the ends are teased. Teasing can be done with a comb or a brush. Try both to determine your preference. Follow these steps to tease the hair:

1. Take a 1-inch section that is 2 ½ inches wide. Hold it between the index and middle fingers and leave a little slack. For finer hair take a smaller section and for thicker hair take a slightly larger section.

2. Insert a comb or brush about 2 to 3 inches away from the scalp.

3. Press the hair toward the scalp in a C formation. Once the hair is pressed toward the scalp, the comb or brush is removed and inserted again. This is repeated 10 to 12 times.

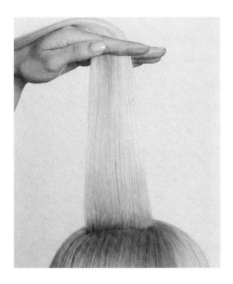 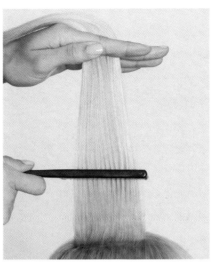 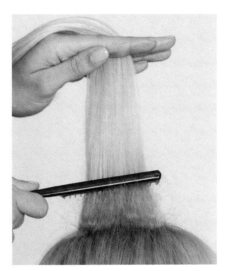

4. Continue with sections of the same size, pressing the hair toward the scalp the same number of times. Tease as close as possible to the previous section for uniform teasing.

5. When teasing to the ends of the hair, complete the cushion near the scalp first. Then insert the comb 3 to 4 inches away from the scalp and press the hair down to meet the other teasing. Keep teasing further and further away from the scalp in a C formation until the ends of the hair are reached.

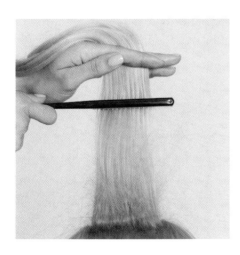 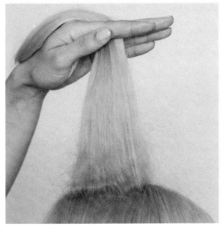

Pinning

Pins are essential for an updo. Without the pins, the updo will not stay in place. The two types of pins used for an updo are bobby pins and hairpins. Pins come in a variety of colors. Pick the appropriate shade for the hair color. Although pins are necessary for an updo, the objective is not to see them.

Bobby pins

Bobby pins are used to hold the hair in place. Open the tip of the pin and slide it along the scalp. Crisscross the pins whenever possible for a secure hold. Bobby pins have rubber tips on the ends for safety. If a pin does not have a rubber tip it should be discarded.

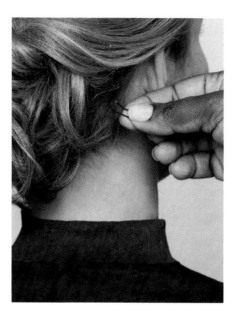 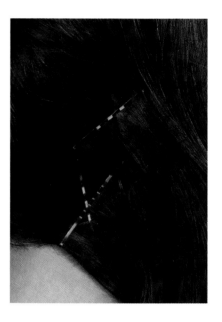

Hairpins

Hairpins are used for the finishing touches on an updo because they are almost invisible—great for pinning the last section or top layer of an updo. Hairpins are also used to hide bobby pins. With the teeth of the hairpin, take about ¼ inch of hair near the bobby pin and cover the bobby pin. Then, slide the hairpin inside the updo.

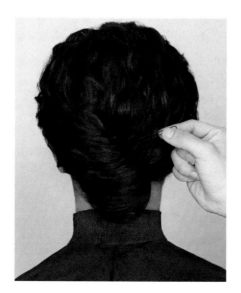 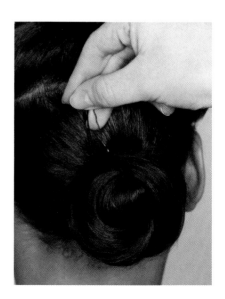

Fillers

Fillers, made from a loose fiber or frizzy hair, are objects that add form, shape, and volume to an updo. They come in a variety of shapes and sizes: doughnut, cylinder, round, and more. The filler should be as close to the client's hair color as possible. Although fillers are not needed for every updo, they are great for adding maximum volume without teasing.

You can also make a filler from a weft of frizzy hair. Choose the amount of hair needed for the filler and then wrap a net around it. The filler is then attached to a flat pin curl. Create a flat pin curl by taking a 1- to 2-inch piece of hair and wrapping it around two fingers near the root area, then flatten the loop on the scalp. Next, crisscross two bobby pins on top of the pin curl. The filler is then bobby pinned into the crisscrossed pins.

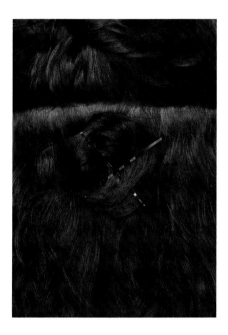 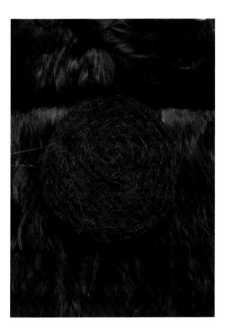

Hair Spray

Hair spray, also known as finishing spray, is the one product used on almost every updo. A light hair spray is needed while constructing the updo. It should be light enough to comb through if a mistake is made. A stronger-hold hair spray is used only when everything is in place. Texture hair sprays, used to achieve a messier finish, are another option. The hair spray container should be held about 10 inches away from the hair. Don't spray directly on the hair; spray above the hair and allow the product to fall down on the hair.

Conclusion

This section discussed the various ways to prepare the hair for an updo. For the purposes of this book, we started with clean hair. Steps for teasing and pinning were also explained. The next sections cover procedures and presents all of the steps for each of the featured hairstyles.

HALF UP

Half up is a great option for women who are unsure about wearing their hair all up. Some clients think they have to wear their hair up for certain occasions. During the consultation, always ask the client if she has worn her hair up before. If the answer is no, this is a good indicator that she might not like her hair all up; you should then suggest a half-up hairstyle. Half up can be as romantic or as edgy as you want it to be.

The following hairstyles have been chosen to show the range of half-up styles: Classic, Sideswept, and Faux Hawk. Adding waves or volume can change each look dramatically.

CLASSIC
HALF UP

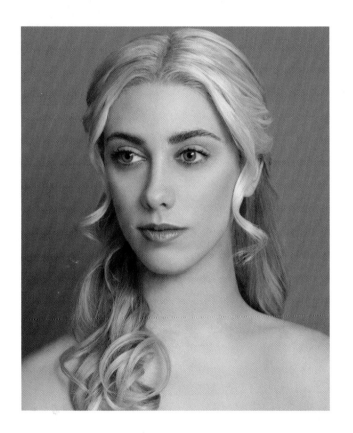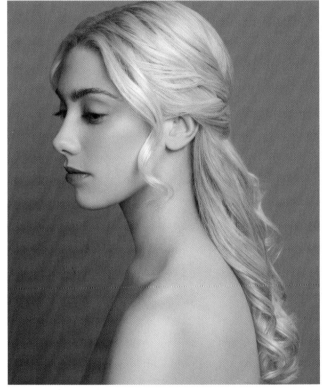

All photos Copyright © 2015 Milady, a part of Cengage Learning®. Photography by Timothy C. Johnson.

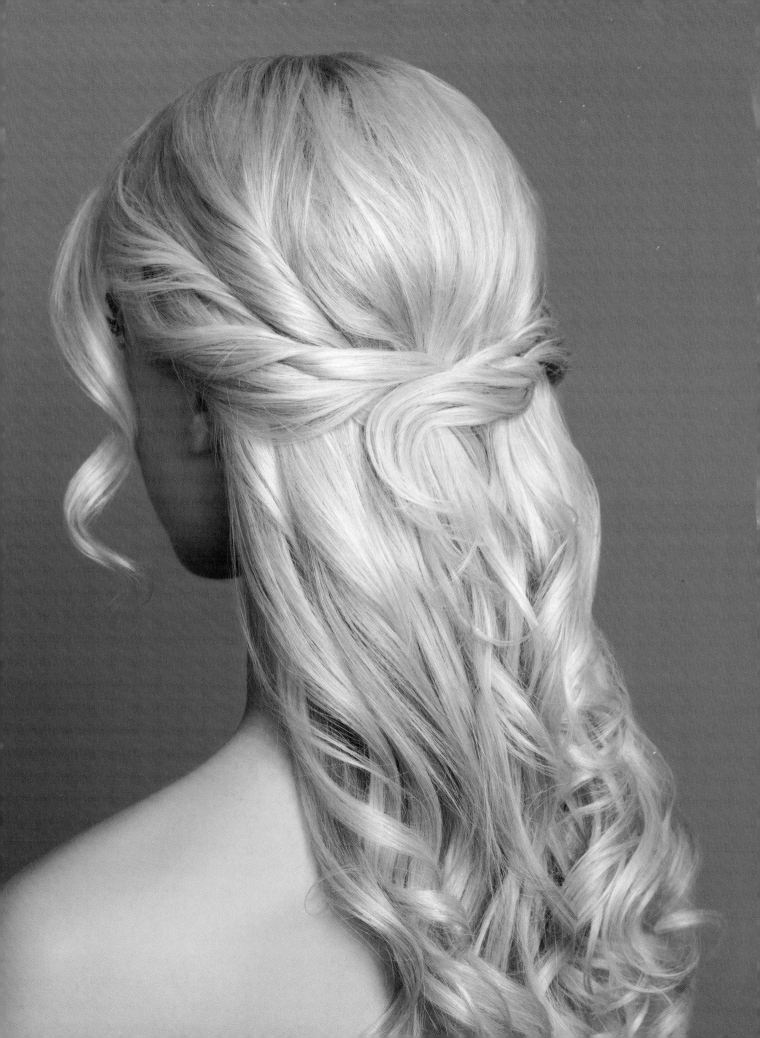

CLASSIC **HALF UP**

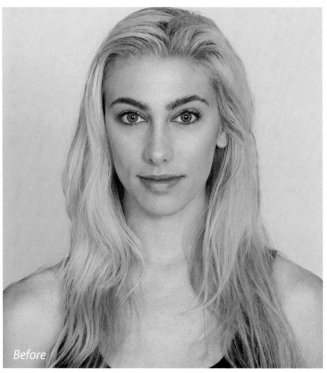

Before

Hair Texture: Fine, Straight
Hair Length: Long

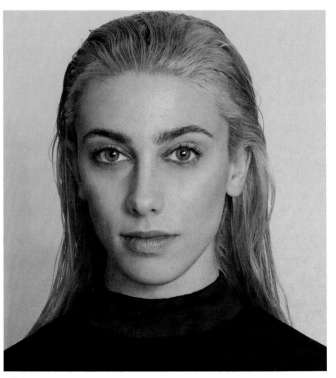

1 Start with hair that has been shampooed and conditioned. Then, apply a styling product best suited for the client's hair type and texture.

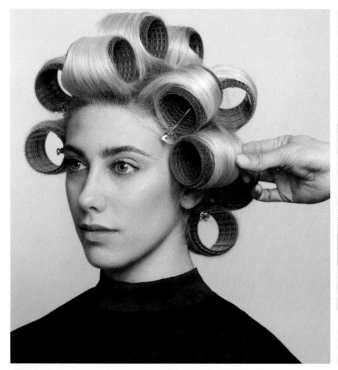

2 Blowdry the hair with a round brush and add rollers while drying the hair for maximum fullness.

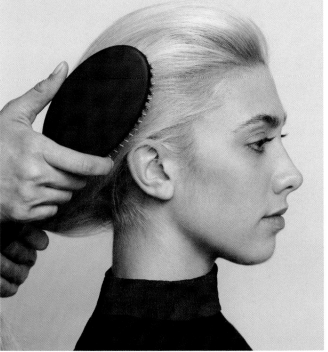

3 Remove the rollers and brush the hair thoroughly to remove all the parts.

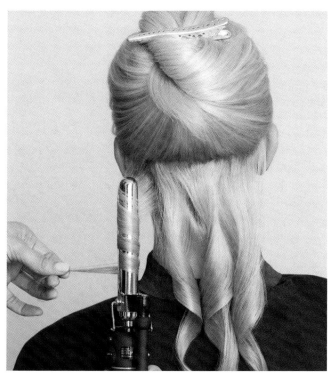

4 Taking vertical sections, curl the hair with a medium-sized curling iron.

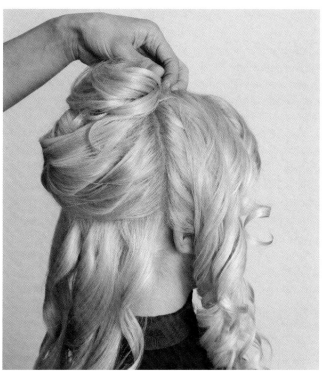

5 Establish a center part using a tail comb. Then, divide the hair into 4 sections: 2 side sections stopping behind the ear, an upper back, and a lower back.

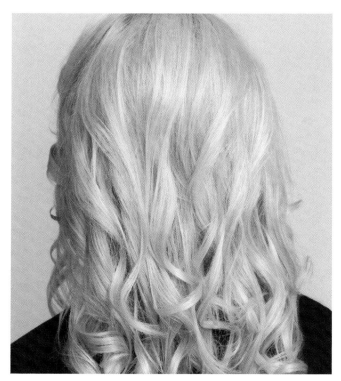

6 Tease the upper-back section and then smooth it into the lower-back section.

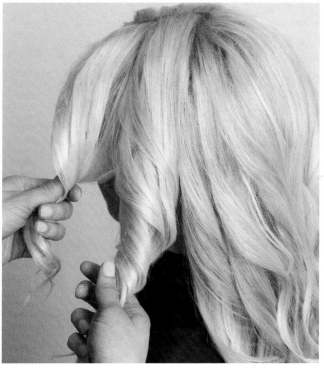

7 Subdivide each side section into 2 sections.

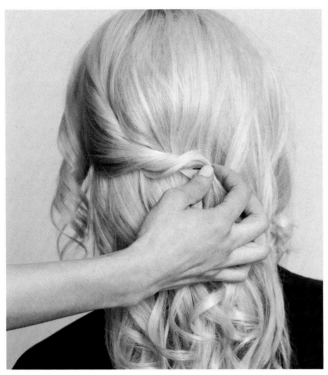

8 Take the left subsection near the ear and twist it. Then, pin it vertically with a bobby pin.

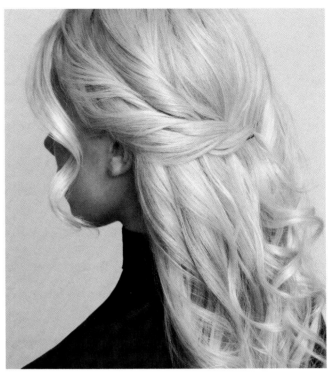

9 Now, take the last subsection and twist it. Then, cross it over the last subsection and pin it vertically. Leave a piece of hair in front to frame the face.

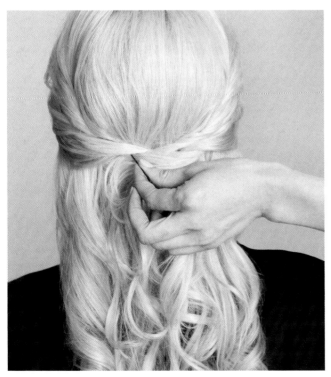

10 Repeat steps 8 and 9 on the right side.

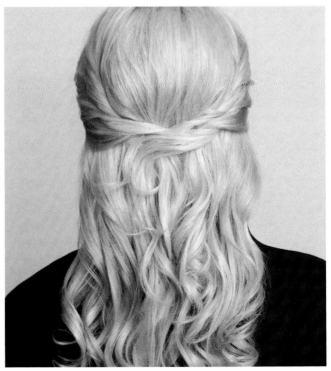

11 Finish with hair spray.

SIDESWEPT
HALF UP

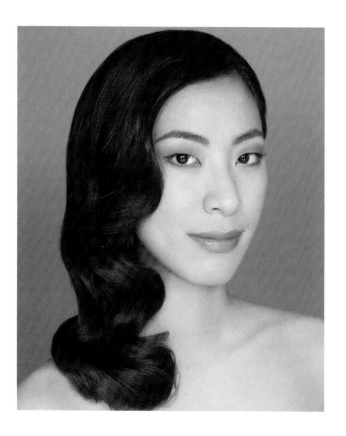
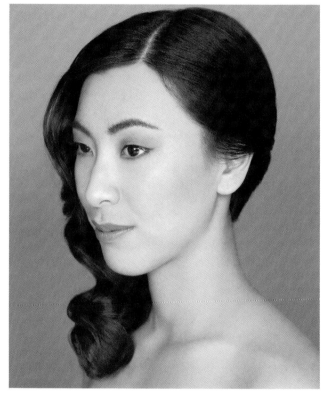

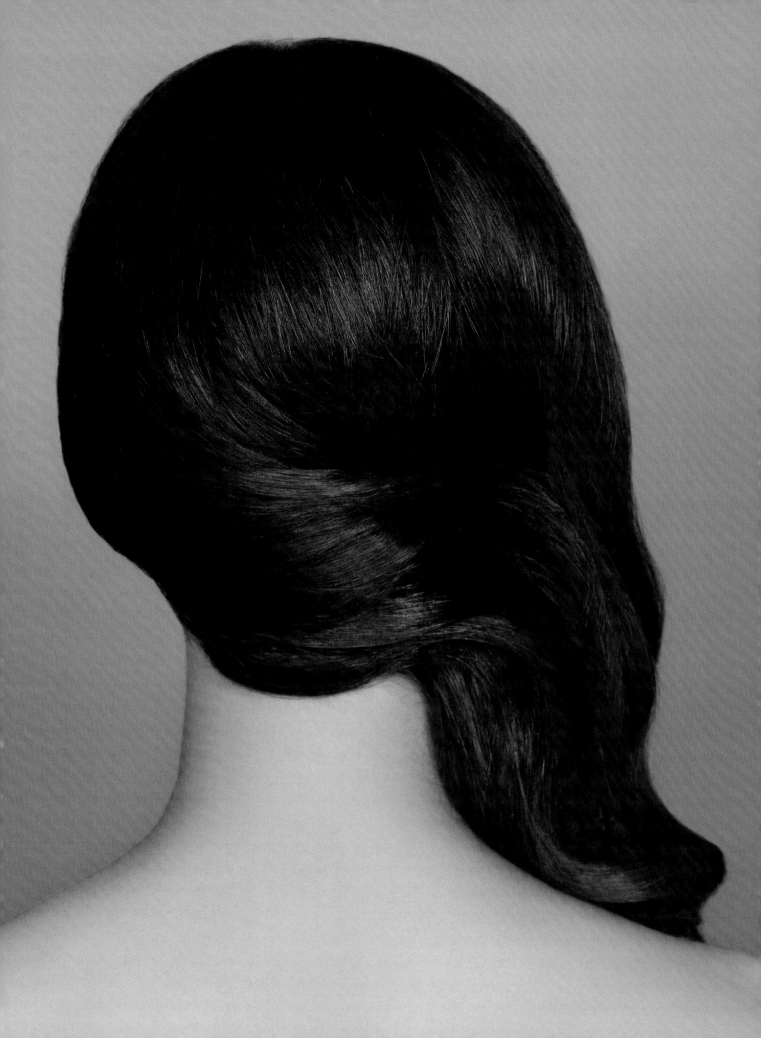

SIDESWEPT HALF UP

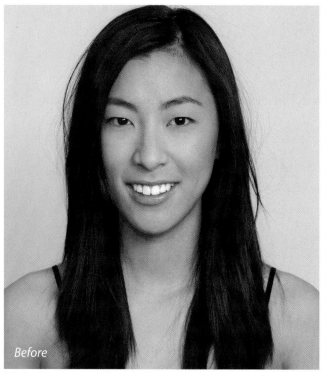

Before

Hair Texture: Straight
Hair Length: Shoulder-length

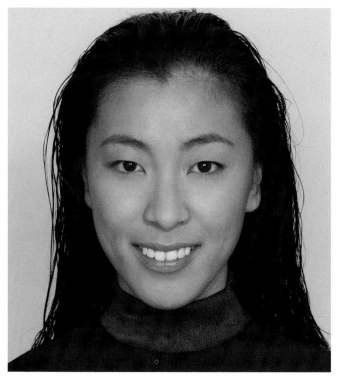

1 Start with hair that has been shampooed and conditioned. Then, apply a styling product best suited for the client's hair type and texture.

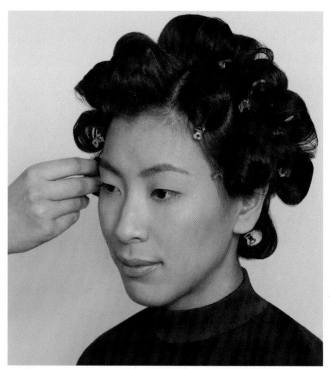

2 Blowdry the hair with a round brush. Then, curl the hair with a medium-sized curling iron and clip each piece for added volume.

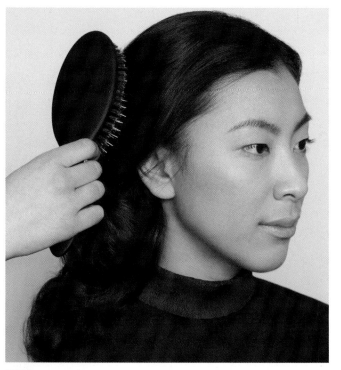

3 Remove the clips and brush the hair thoroughly to remove all the parts.

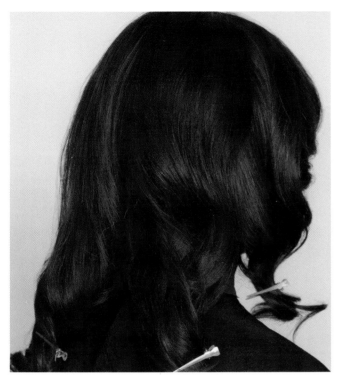

4 Establish a side part. Then, divide the hair into 4 sections. Separate the hair from above the apex to behind the ear and split the hair down the center in the back.

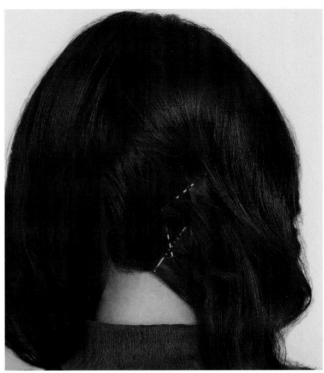

5 Starting with the right back section, direct the hair to the right about 1 inch and create a base with a row of crisscrossed bobby pins.

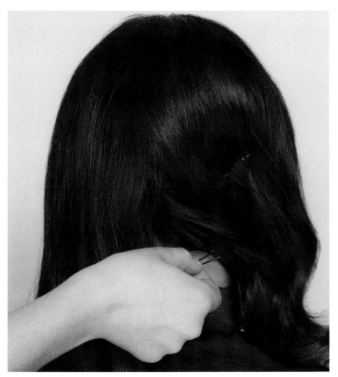

6 Divide the left back section into 3 to 4 subsections. Twist the first section and pin with hairpins into the base of the crisscrossed pins.

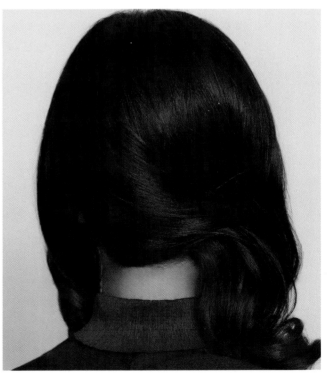

7 Continue to twist and pin until the back section is completed.

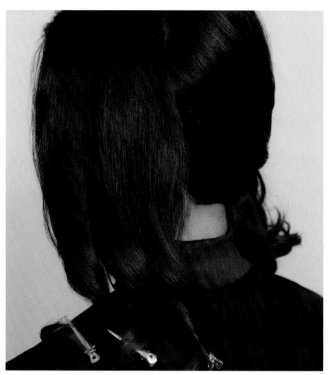

8 The left side section is then divided into 3 subsections.

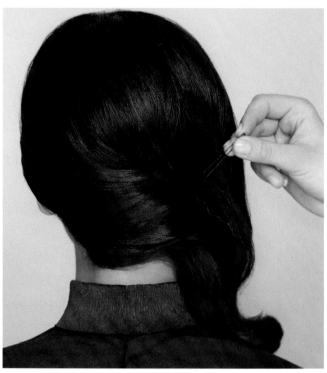

9 Twist and pin each piece on top of the other section.

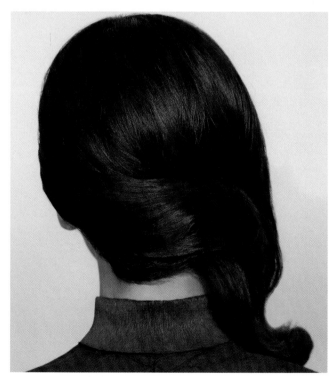

10 Finish with hair spray.

FAUX HAWK
HALF UP

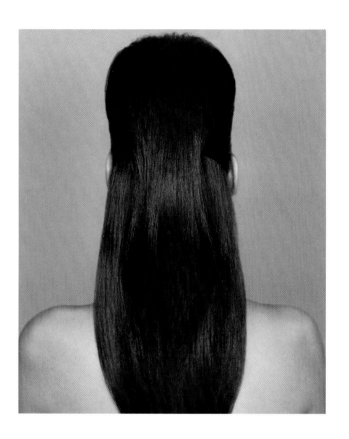

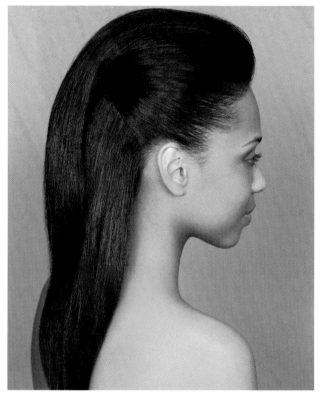

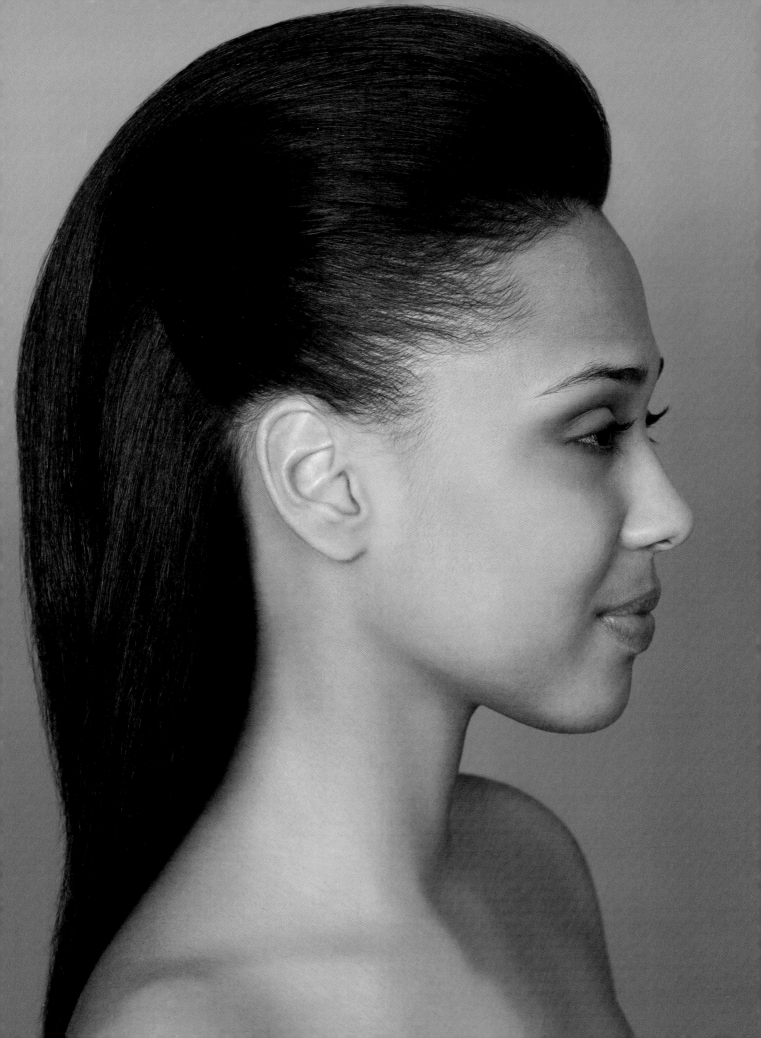

FAUX HAWK **HALF UP**

Before

Hair Texture: Curly
Hair Length: Long

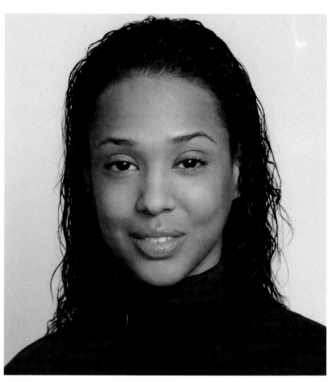

1 Start with hair that has been shampooed and conditioned. Then, apply a styling product best suited for the client's hair type and texture.

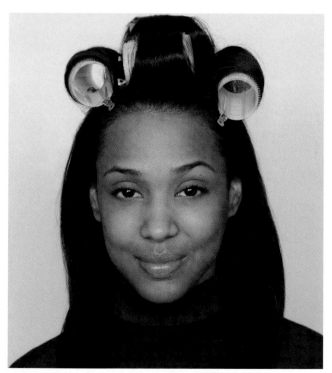

2 Blowdry the hair with a round brush. Then, curl the top with a large curling iron and add rollers. Smooth the remaining hair with a flat iron.

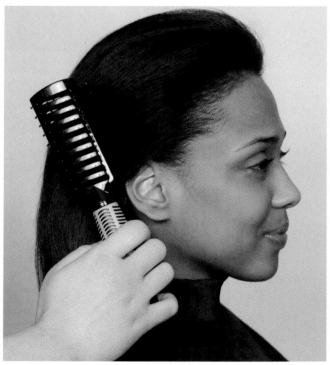

3 Remove the rollers and brush the hair thoroughly to remove all the parts.

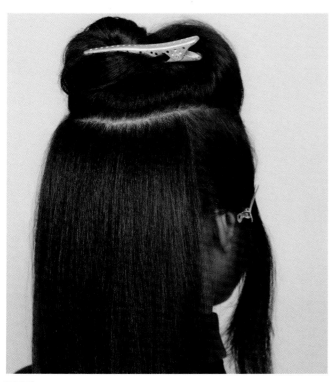

4 Divide the hair into 4 sections. Section off the crown from temple to temple and from the forehead to 3 inches below the apex. The side sections are divided just behind the ear and the back section is left hanging.

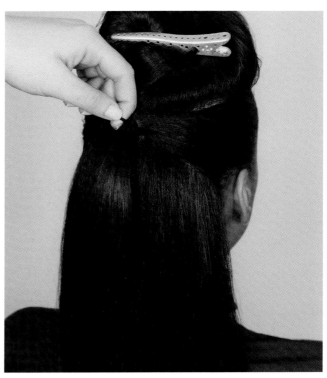

5 Take both sides and brush them back tightly with a cushion brush and secure with an elastic band 3 to 4 inches below the apex.

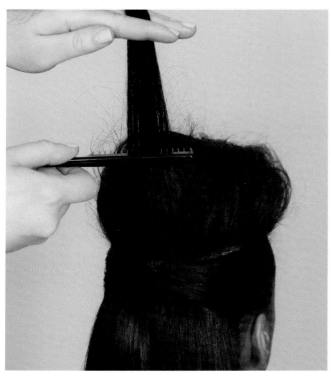

6 Tease the entire crown and apply hair spray.

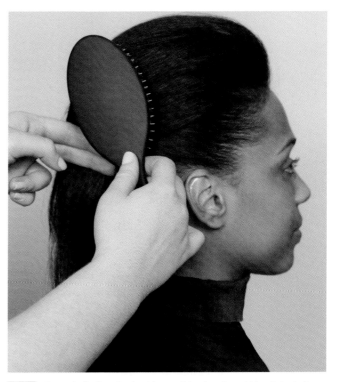

7 Smooth the hair back with a cushion brush and blend the hair with the sides. The top should be about 2 to 3 inches high.

Faux Hawk Half Up   **27**

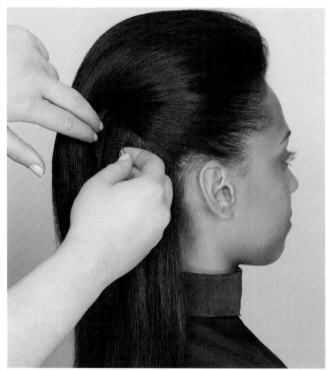

8 Pin the top and sides toward the elastic band.

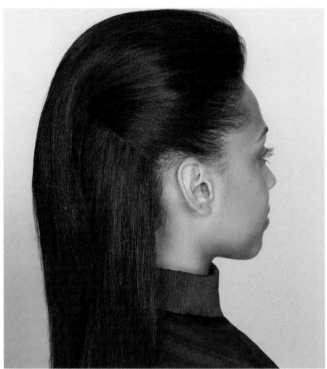

9 Finish with hair spray.

PONYTAIL

Nearly everyone has worn a ponytail at one time or another—it is the go-to hairstyle for many women. But, do not underestimate the beauty of the ponytail. When the texture is refined or volume added, a ponytail is quite stunning. Some women just feel prettier with some of their hair down, and a polished ponytail is the perfect choice.

Ponytail with Volume has an added weft of hair to elongate the hair. Ponytail with Detail has been done in a more intricate way. Finally, Ponytail Hawk has volume and a unique way of being held in place. Whether sleek or with added volume, the ponytail is timeless.

PONYTAIL
WITH VOLUME

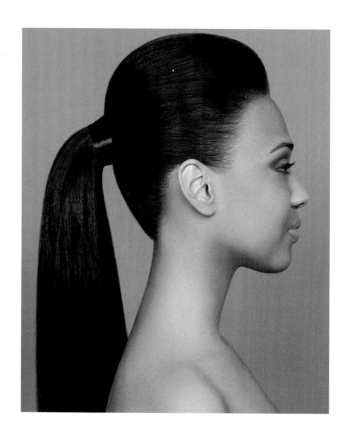
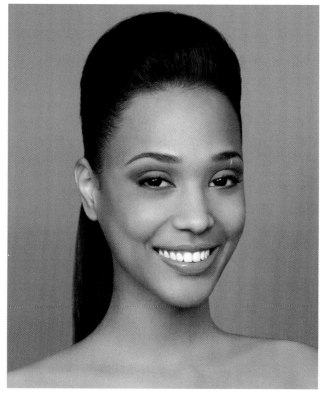

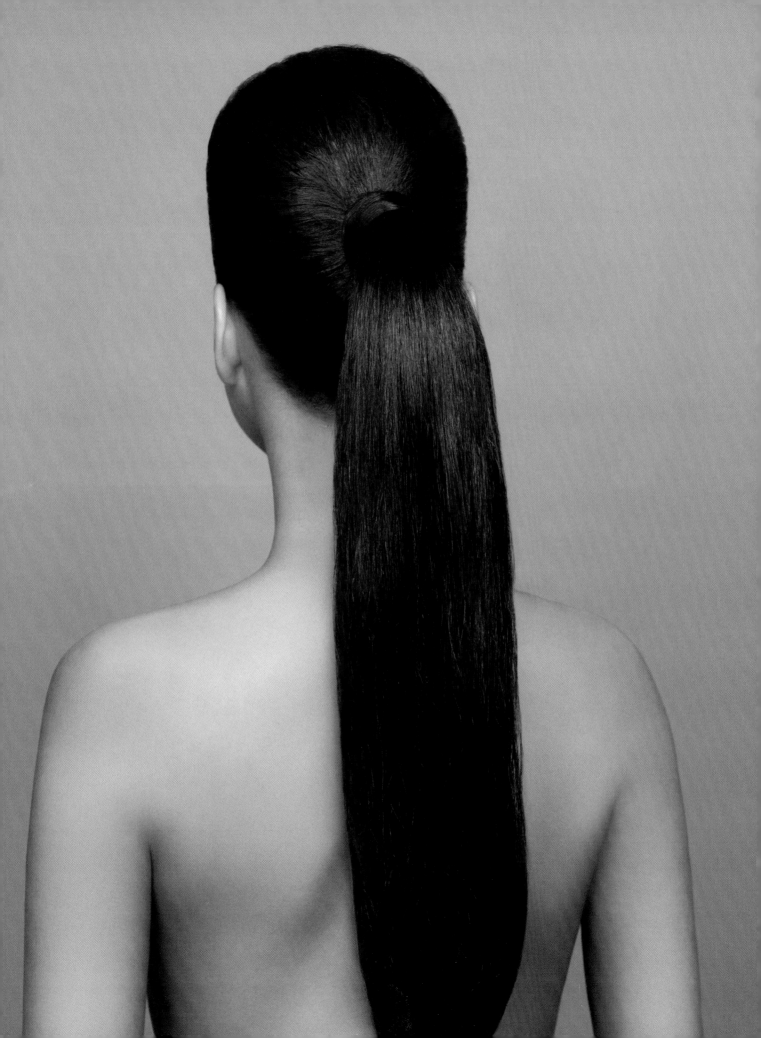

PONYTAIL **WITH VOLUME**

Before

Hair Texture: Curly
Hair Length: Long

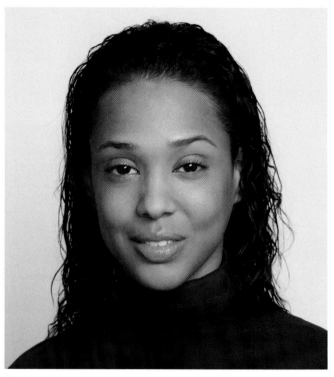

1 Start with hair that has been shampooed and conditioned. Then, apply a styling product best suited for the client's hair type and texture.

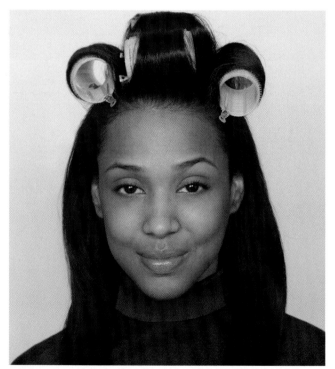

2 Blowdry the hair with a round brush. Then, smooth the top with a large curling iron and add rollers. Smooth the remaining hair with a flat iron.

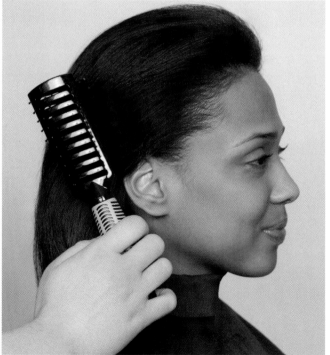

3 Remove the rollers and brush the hair thoroughly to remove all the parts.

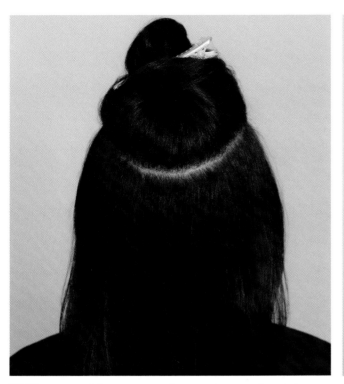

4 Section off the entire crown from temple to temple and about 3 inches below the apex.

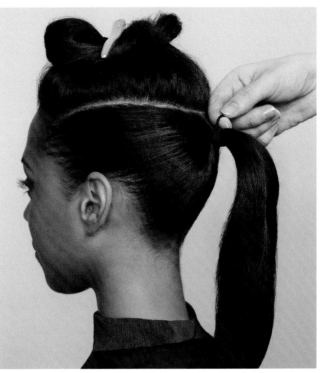

5 Brush the hair with a cushion brush into a ponytail with an elastic band just above the occipital bone. Make sure the ponytail is centered.

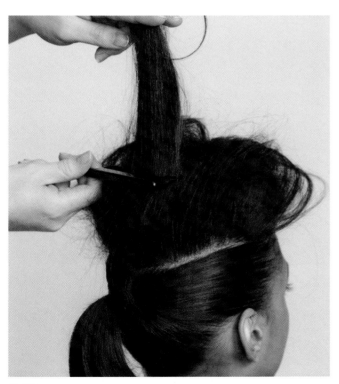

6 Tease the entire crown section and lightly use hair spray.

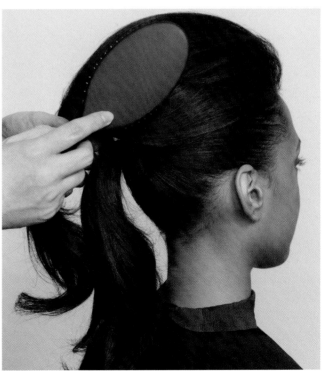

7 Smooth the hair back with a cushion brush, leaving it about 2 to 3 inches in height.

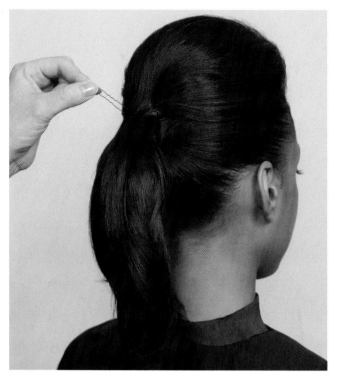

8 Blend the top hair in with the sides using a cushion brush and pin the hair to the top of the ponytail with hairpins. Use hair spray as needed.

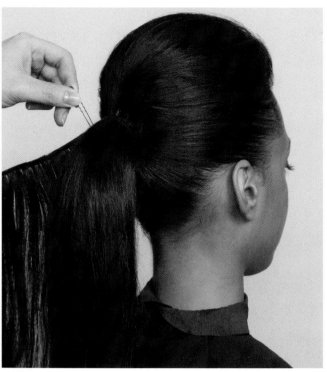

9 Attach human hair on a weft by wrapping it around the elastic band and pinning with hairpins as you go. You will later bend the pins if they are visible. Wrap the hair until the shorter ponytail is hidden.

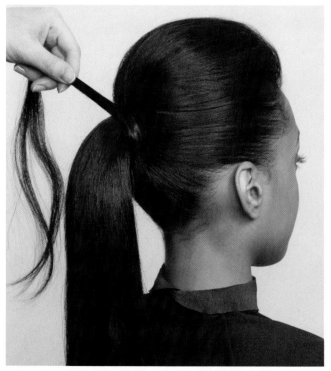

10 Take a piece of the hair and wrap it around the elastic band and secure with hairpins.

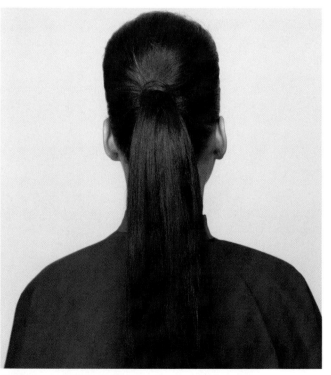

11 Finish with hair spray.

PONYTAIL
WITH DETAIL

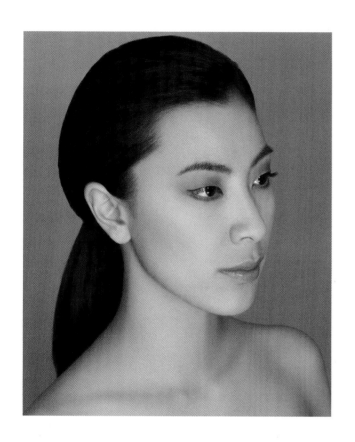 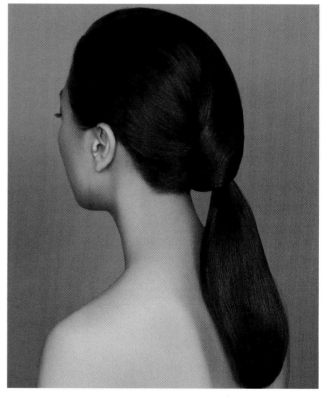

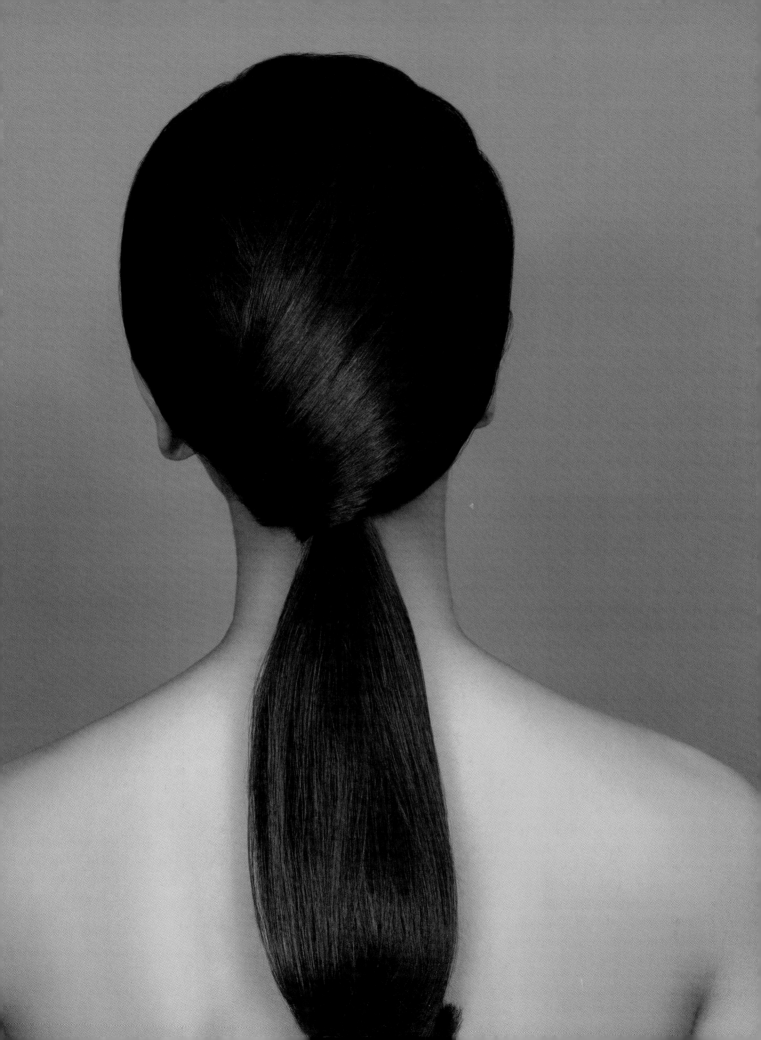

PONYTAIL **WITH DETAIL**

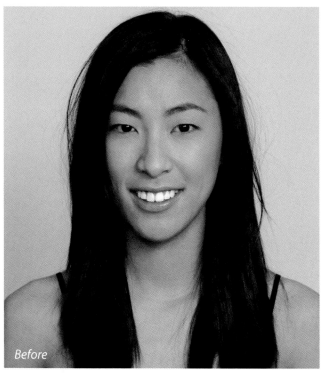

Before

Hair Texture: Straight
Hair Length: Shoulder-length

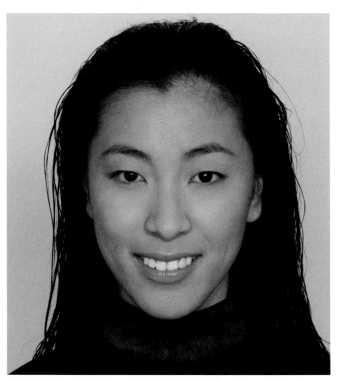

1 Start with hair that has been shampooed and conditioned. Then, apply a styling product best suited for the client's hair type and texture.

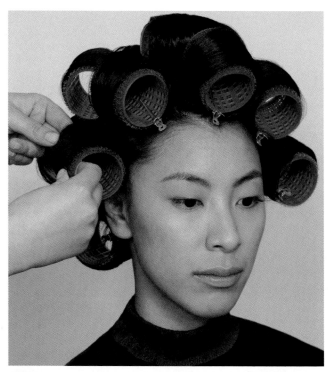

2 Blowdry the hair with a round brush and add rollers while drying the hair for maximum fullness.

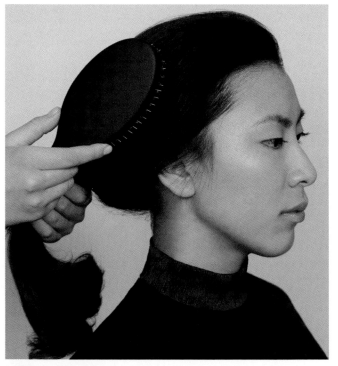

3 Remove the rollers and brush the hair thoroughly to remove all the parts.

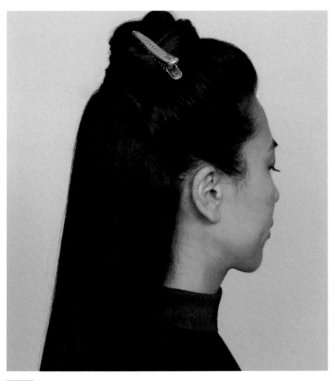

4 Divide the hair into 2 sections, front and back, from behind the ear and just behind the apex.

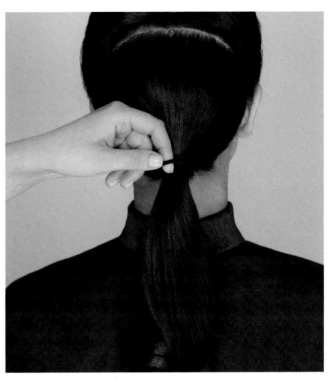

5 Gather the back section into a low ponytail with an elastic band, 1 inch above the back hairline and centered.

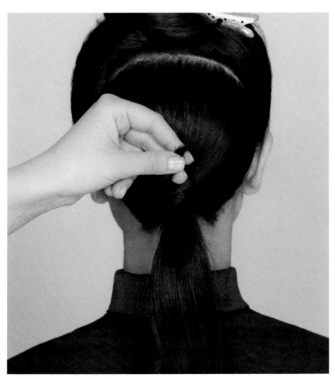

6 Wrap a small piece of hair around the elastic band and secure with bobby pins.

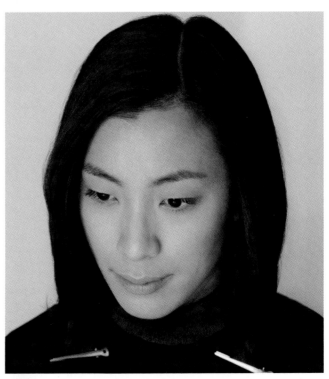

7 Establish a side parting and divide it into 2 sections.

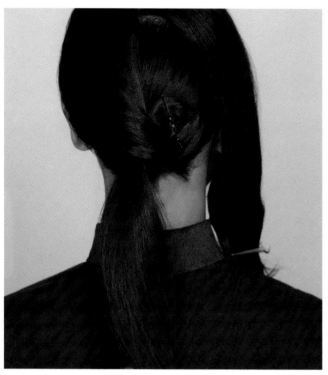

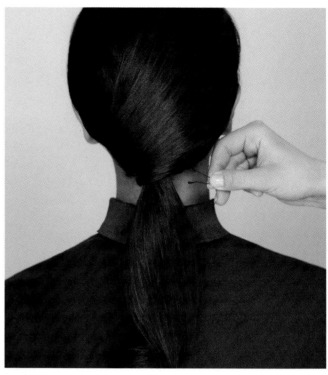

8 Using your fingers, take the side with less hair, pull it back, and direct it over to the opposite side of the ponytail. Make a flat pin curl with the ends of the hair and crisscross two bobby pins to secure.

9 Using your fingers, take the heavier side, cross it over the last section, and wrap it around the ponytail. Tuck the hair underneath and secure with bobby pins.

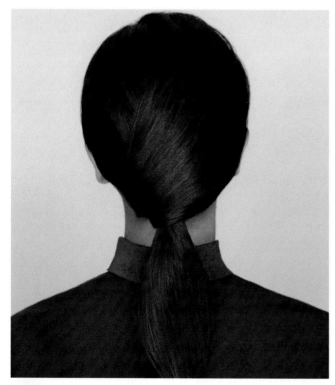

10 Finish with hair spray.

PONYTAIL HAWK

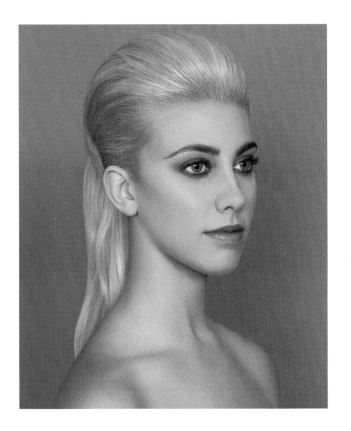 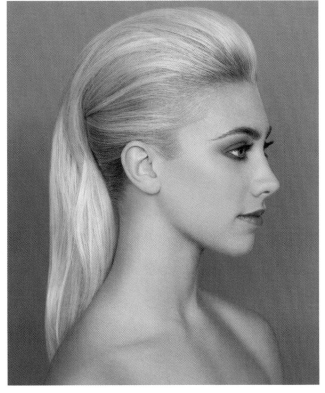

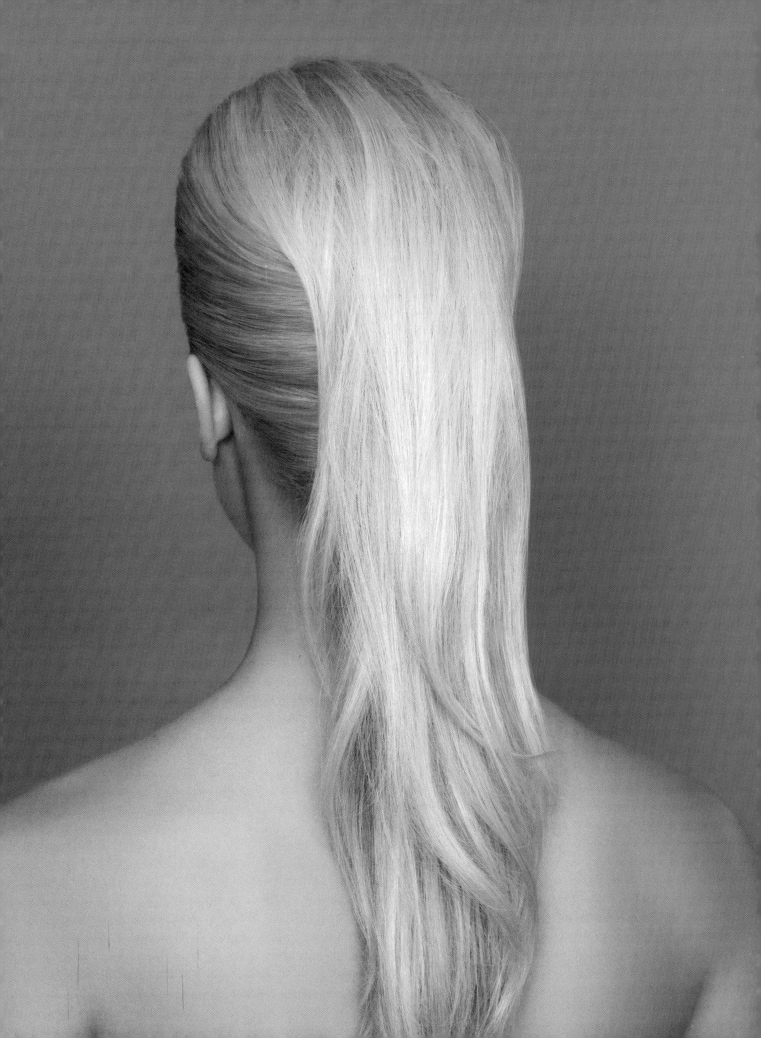

PONYTAIL **HAWK**

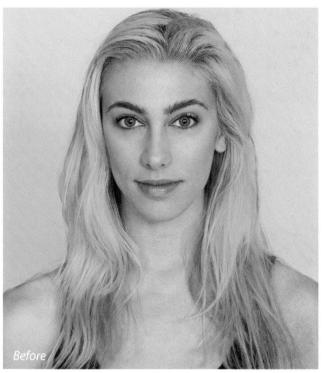

Before

Hair Texture: Fine, straight
Hair Length: Long

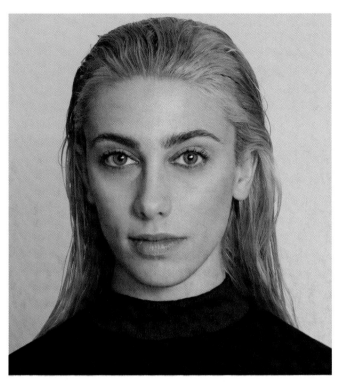

1 Start with hair that has been shampooed and conditioned. Then, apply a styling product best suited for the client's hair type and texture.

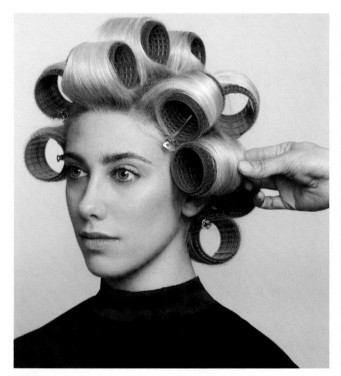

2 Blowdry the hair with a medium-sized round brush and add rollers while drying the hair for maximum fullness.

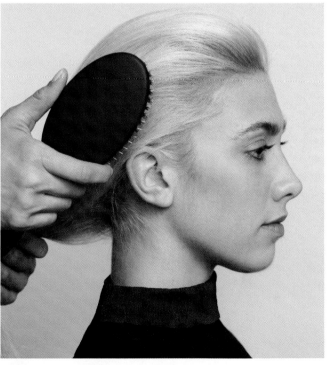

3 Remove the rollers and brush the hair thoroughly to remove all the parts.

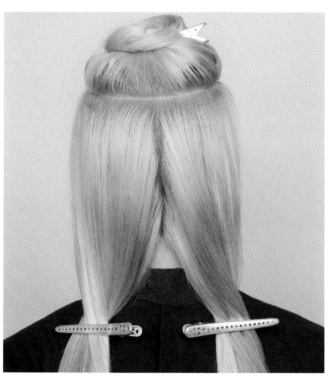

4 Divide the hair into 3 sections. The crown section goes from temple to temple and stops 2 inches below the apex; then split the hair down the center of the back to make the last 2 sections.

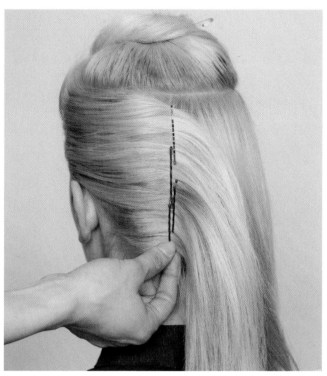

5 Brush the left side section toward the middle of the back with a cushion brush. Pin it on top of the hair in a vertical row with the bobby pins about 1 inch to the left of center.

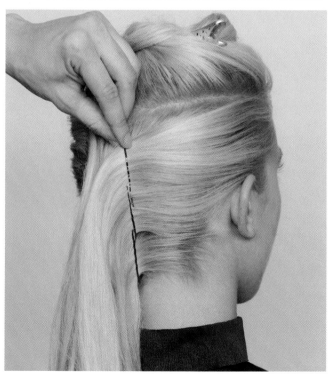

6 Brush the right side section toward the middle of the back with a cushion brush. Pin it on top of the hair in a vertical row with bobby pins about 1 inch to the right of center.

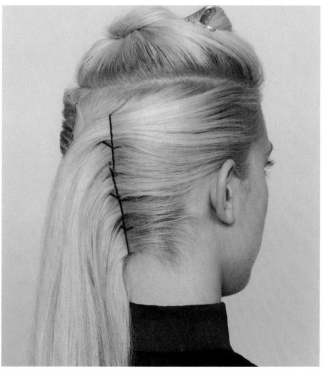

7 Make sure the back is centered. Then, crisscross each pin at an angle up on both sides.

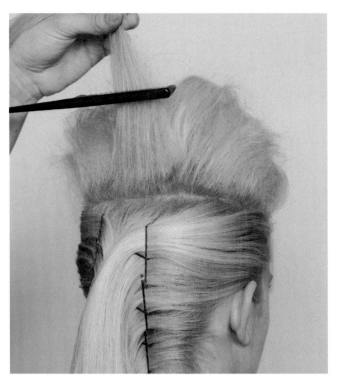

8 Tease the crown section with a teasing comb.

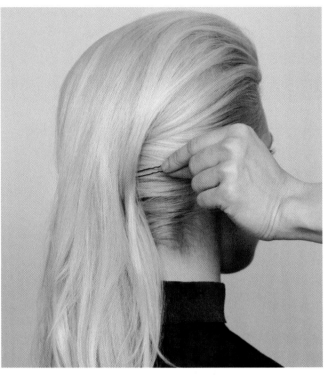

9 Smooth the crown section toward the center of the back with a cushion brush and use hairpins to secure.

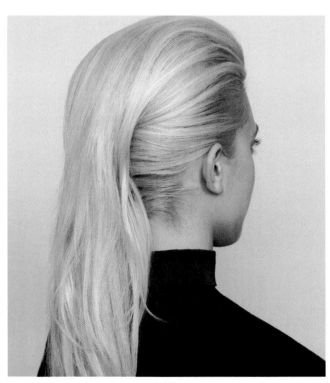

10 Finish with hair spray.

CHIGNON

The chignon is one of the most popular updos. Many famous women have worn this hairstyle, including Diana Ross, Eva Peron, Sara Jessica Parker, Jennifer Lopez, and the list goes on. It is a very elegant hairstyle but it can also be edgy.

Here we demonstrate the Classic, Messy, and Side Chignon. It really depends on the personality of the client which choice is made. A filler was added to the Classic Chignon for fullness. With the help of fillers and hairpieces, the chignon can be as large as you like. The Messy Chignon is more playful for those who want a "done but undone" look. The Side Chignon has been constructed in a more intricate way for added detail. Leaving hair around the face softens the look.

CLASSIC
CHIGNON

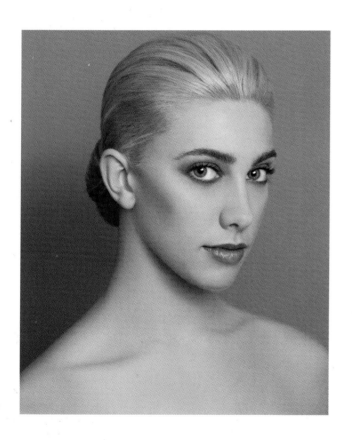
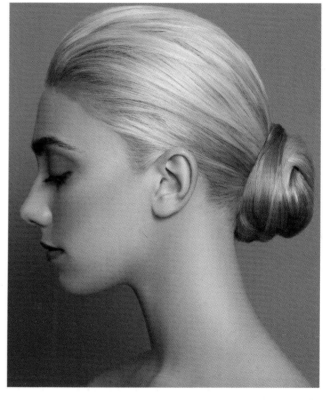

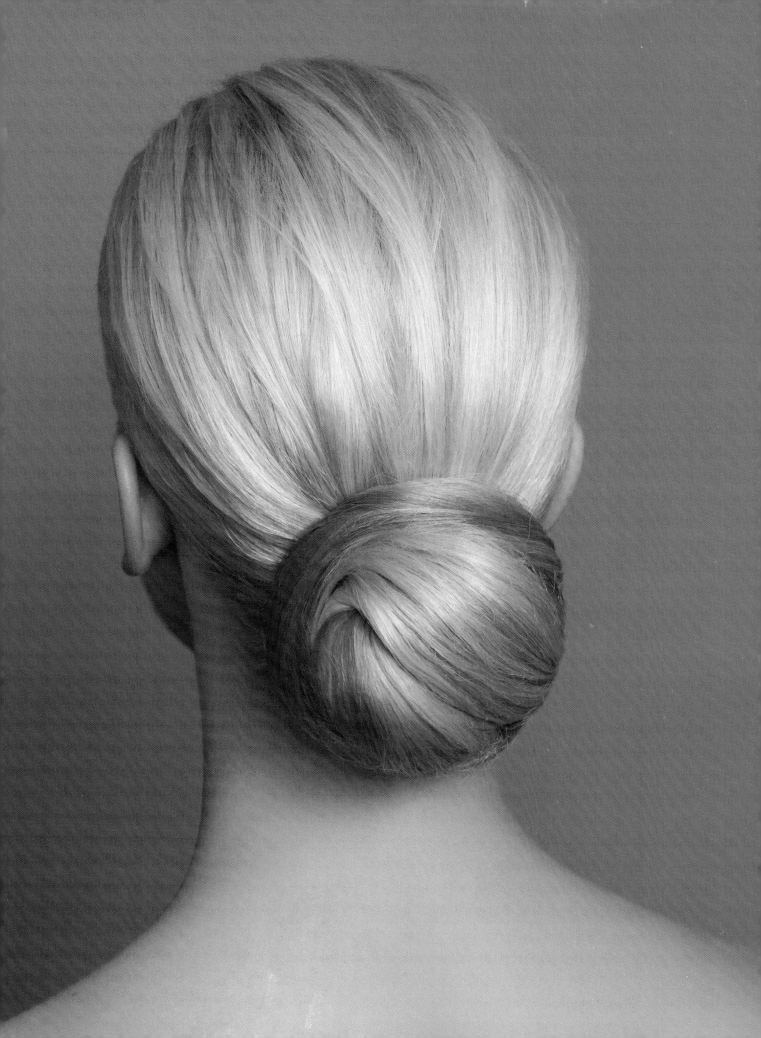

CLASSIC CHIGNON

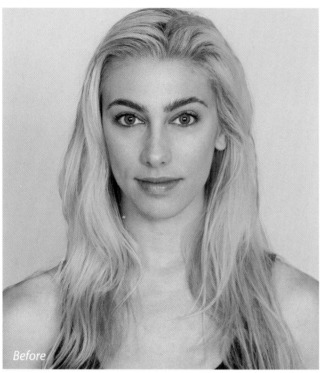

Before

Hair Texture: Fine, straight
Hair Length: Shoulder-length

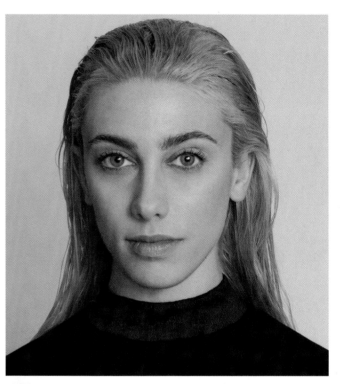

1 Start with hair that has been shampooed, conditioned, and towel-dried. Apply a styling product best suited for the client's hair type and texture.

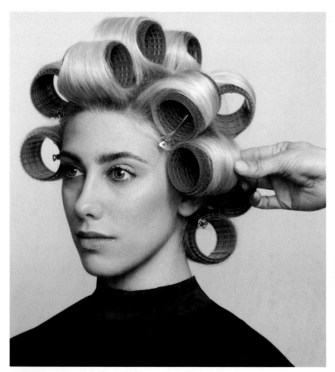

2 Take 2 ½-inch sections and blowdry the hair, adding body with a medium-sized round brush, and add rollers while drying the hair for maximum fullness.

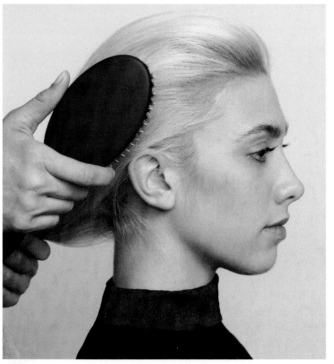

3 Take the rollers out and brush the hair until all parts have disappeared.

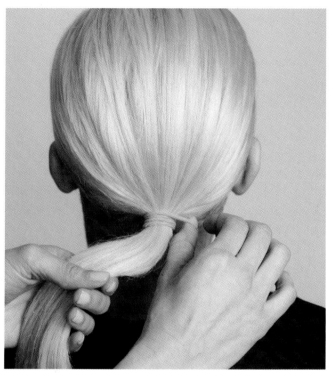

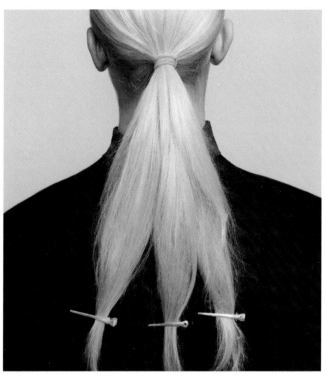

4 Brush the hair back with a cushion brush and then run your fingers through it for added texture. Secure the hair with an elastic band about 1 inch from the back hairline, centered. Use hair spray for the flyaways.

5 Tease the loose hair and divide it into 3 sections.

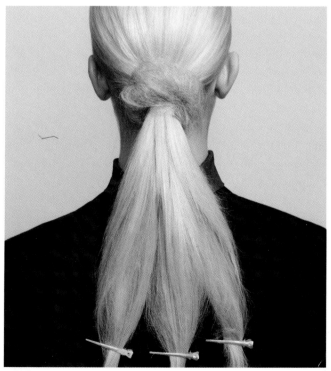

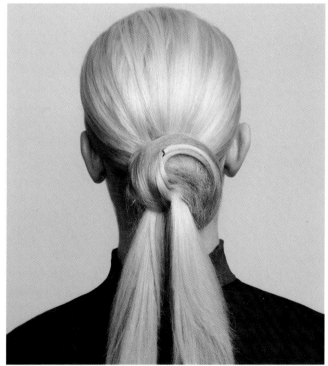

6 Wrap a small, teased weft of hair around the elastic and secure with bobby pins. Make sure the weft of hair is a close match to the client's hair color.

7 Smooth the top layer of the middle piece with a cushion brush and pin around the weft of hair clockwise. Add hair spray as needed.

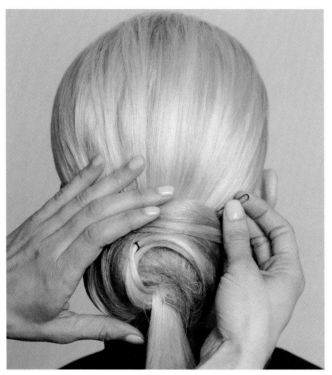

8 The left piece of the loose hair is pinned clockwise.

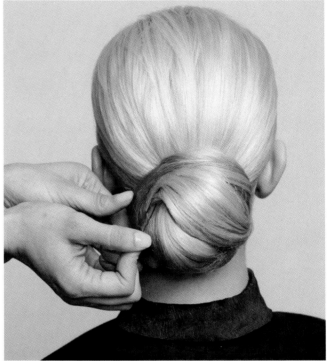

9 The last piece is first pinned counterclockwise and then directed clockwise, being careful not to show any gaps. A combination of bobby pins and hairpins should be used on this section.

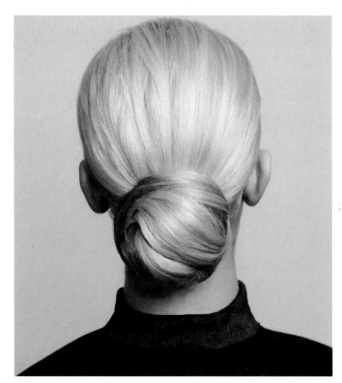

10 Finish the look with hair spray.

MESSY CHIGNON

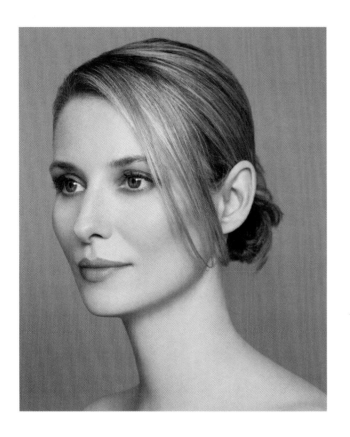
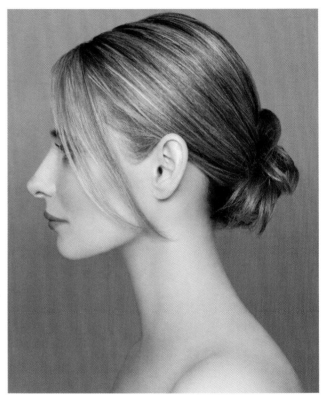

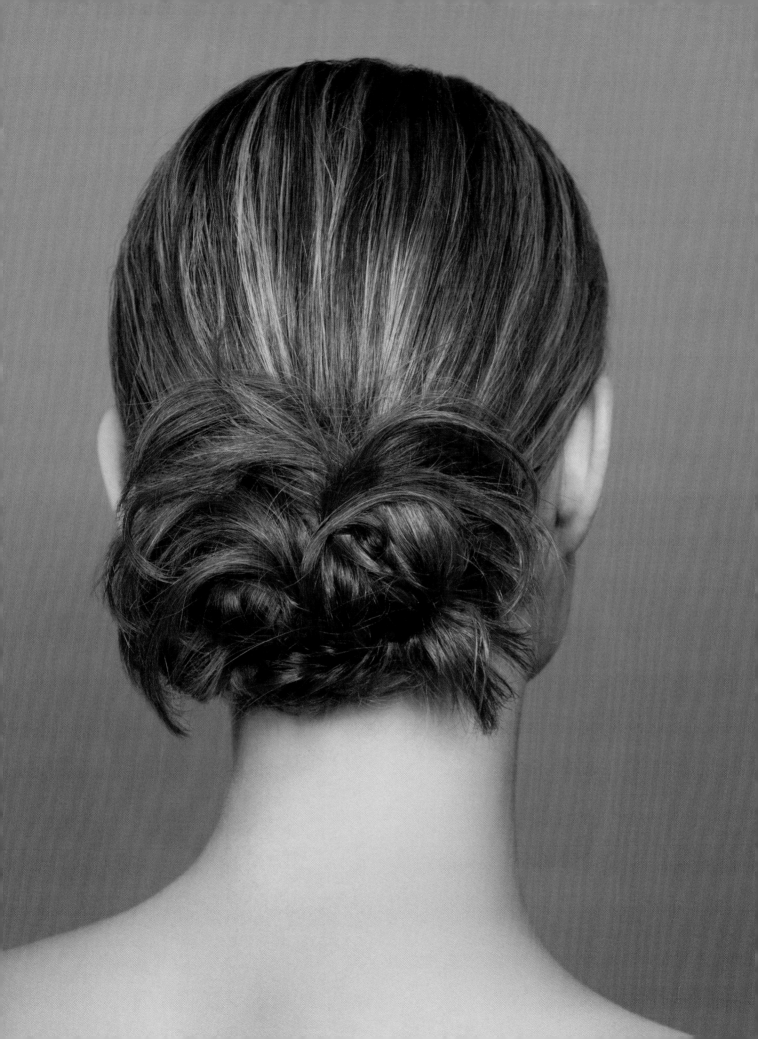

MESSY CHIGNON

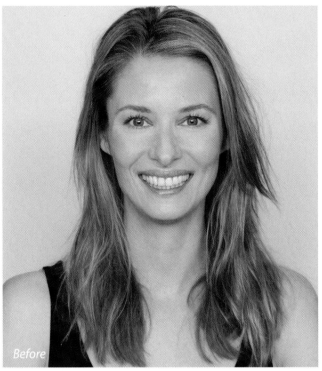

Hair Texture: Straight
Hair Length: Shoulder-length

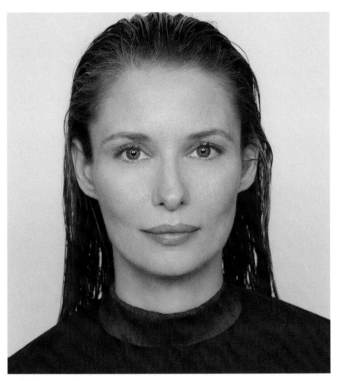

1 Start with hair that has been shampooed and conditioned. Apply a styling product best suited for the client's hair type and texture.

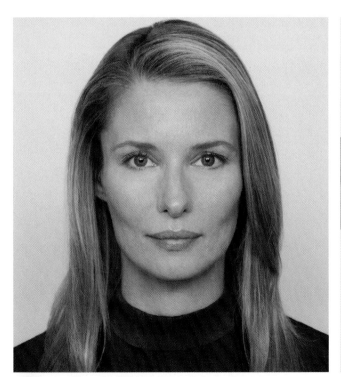

2 Blowdry the hair, adding body with a round brush.

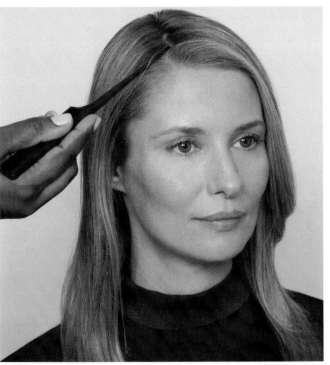

3 Create a zigzag part on the side by using the end of a tail comb.

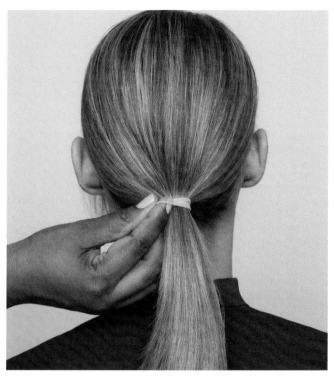

4 Leave a few pieces out around the face for softness and direct back with fingers. Secure with an elastic band about 1½ inches above the hairline.

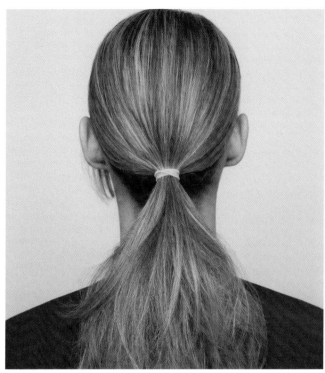

5 Tease the loose hair slightly and apply texture spray.

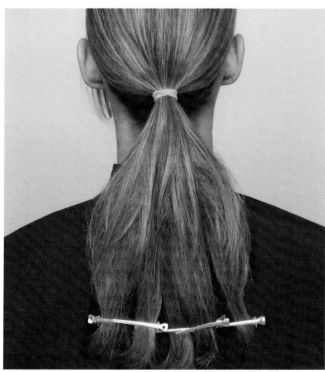

6 Divide the hair into 5 to 6 sections.

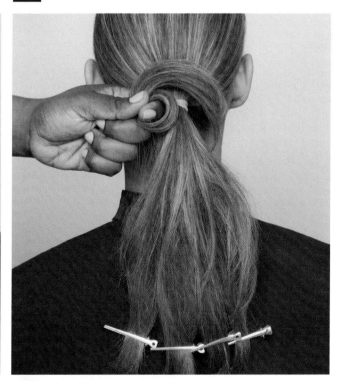

7 Starting near the scalp, loop a section around your finger and leave about 3 inches of the ends out. Then, pin the loop toward the elastic band with bobby pins. If the hair is very long it can be looped twice. Crisscross the pins to make the updo secure.

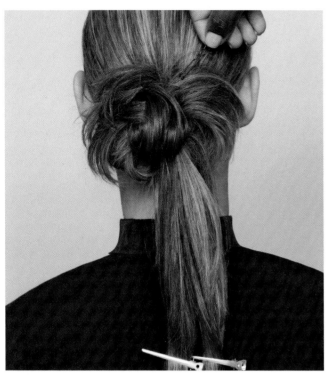

8 Moving clockwise, repeat step 7. The ends sticking out should be placed on the side and top of the chignon. Also, the loops can be slightly irregular.

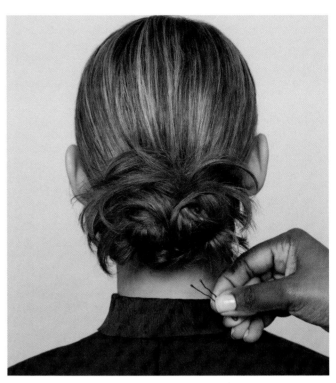

9 The last 2 sections should be pinned toward the elastic band while allowing the loose hair to stick out through the center.

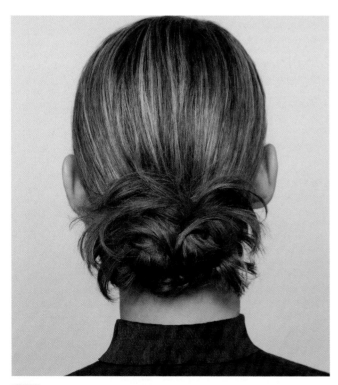

10 Finish with texture spray.

SIDE
CHIGNON

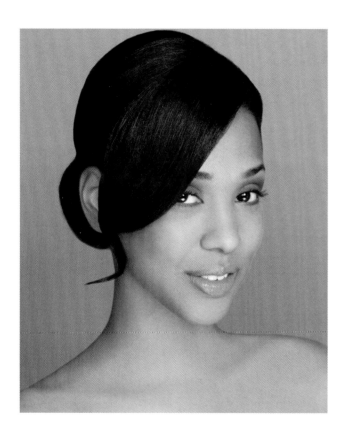
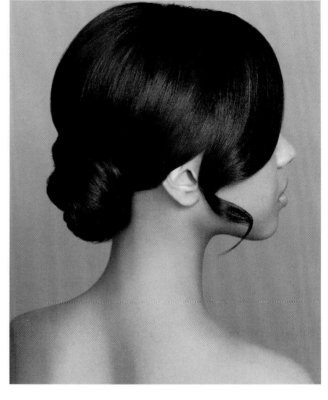

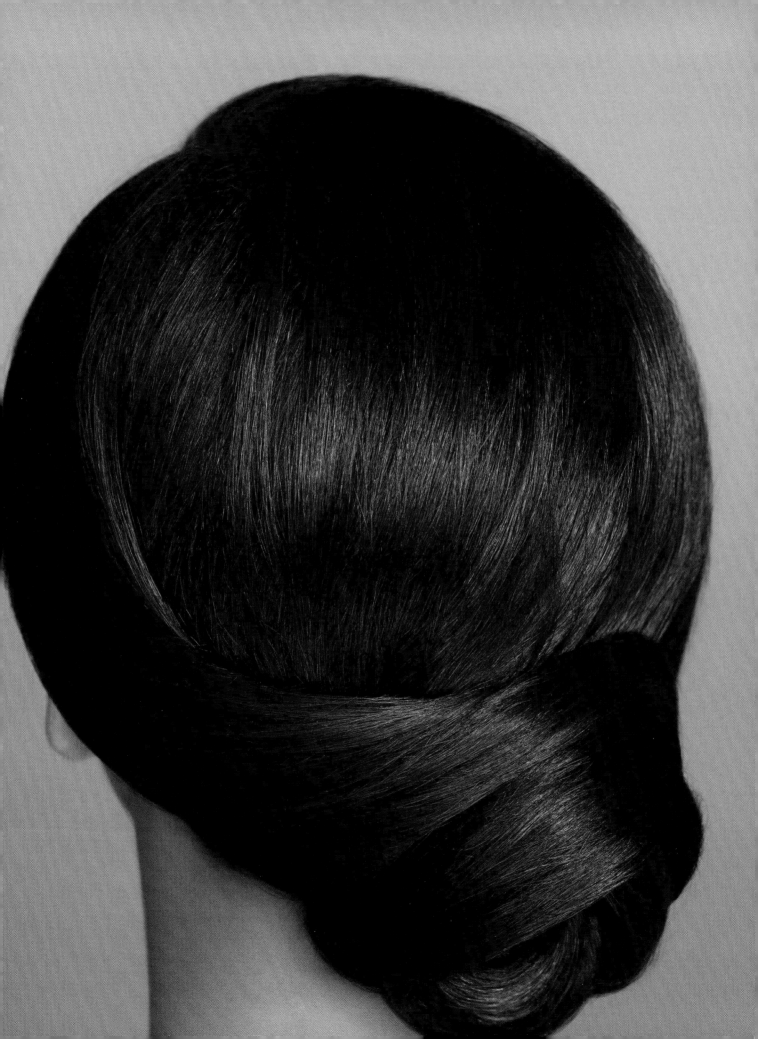

SIDE **CHIGNON**

Before

Hair Texture: Curly
Hair Length: Long

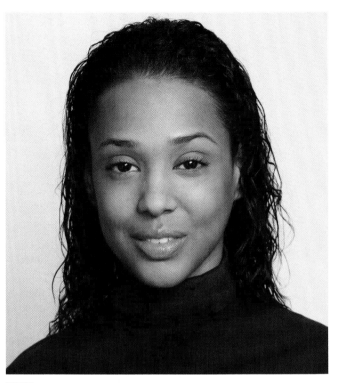

1 Start with hair that has been shampooed and conditioned. Apply styling products best suited for the client's hair type and texture.

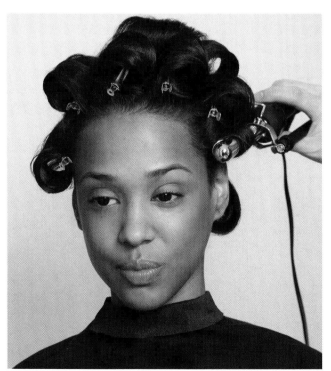

2 Blowdry the hair straight, adding body with a round brush. Then, curl the hair with a medium-sized curling iron and clip each piece.

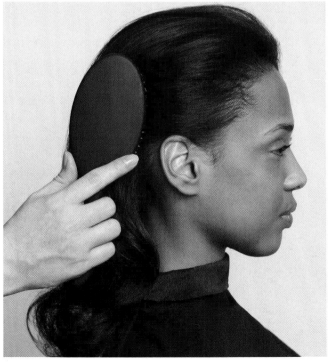

3 Remove the clips and brush the hair well to eliminate the parts.

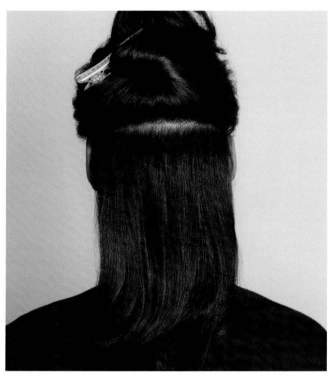

4 Using the end of a tail comb, make a part from ear to ear and put the top section in a clip.

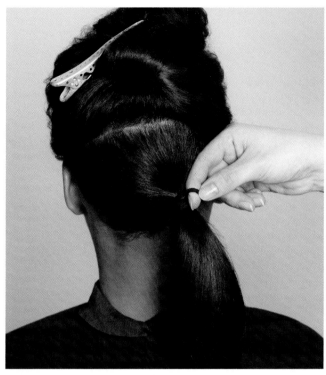

5 Direct the back section to the right side of the head and secure the hair with an elastic band, 1 inch above the back hairline and 1 inch from the side.

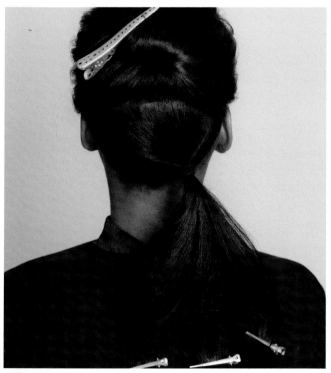

6 Tease the hair and mist with a light hair spray. Then, divide the hair into 3 sections.

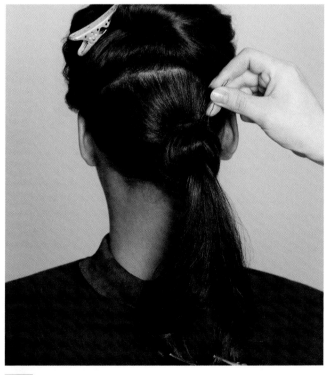

7 Starting with the left piece, wrap the section loosely around the elastic band clockwise and pin with bobby pins while wrapping.

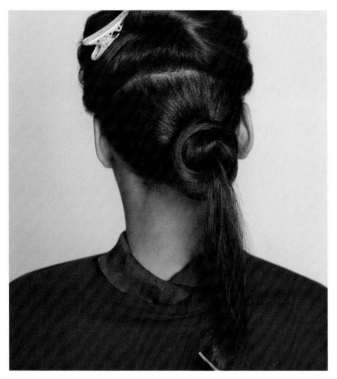

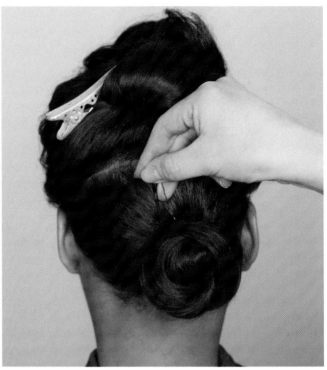

8 Take the next section and pin it around the first section in the same direction, being careful not to wrap it too tight.

9 The last section should be wrapped the same as described in step 8 and secure with bobby pins.

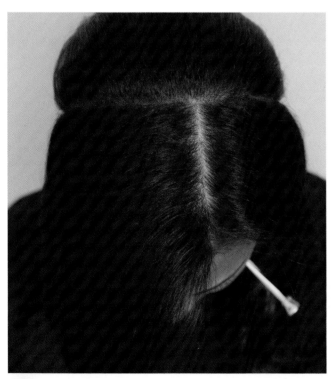

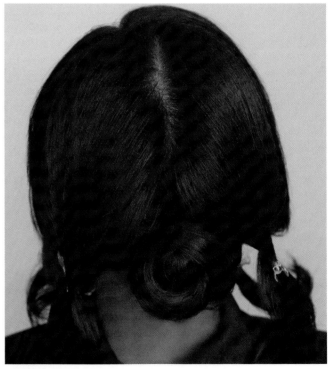

10 Take the clipped hair down and add a side part on the opposite side of the chignon. Then, divide the hair into 3 sections: 1 back section and 2 side sections.

11 Divide the back into 2 sections.

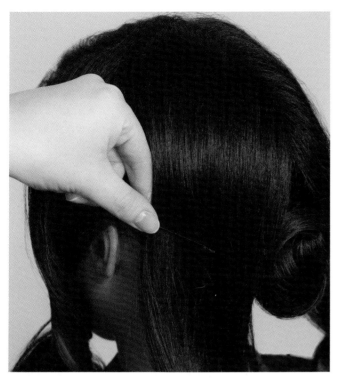

12 Position the bobby pins diagonally from the top of the ear toward the chignon on the left back section.

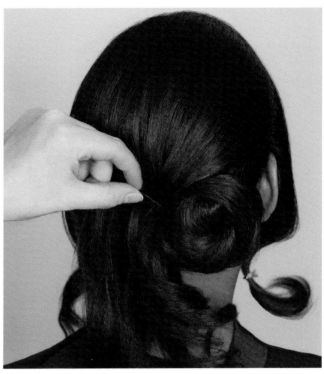

13 Split the right back section in 2 pieces and direct those pieces over to the previous section, one at a time, and pin. Allow this hair to remain loose.

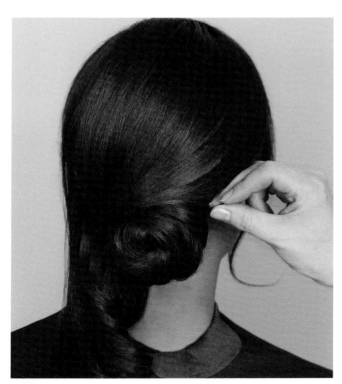

14 Take the right side section and direct it to the left side of the chignon and pin it around the chignon counterclockwise. Leave a piece of hair around the face for softness.

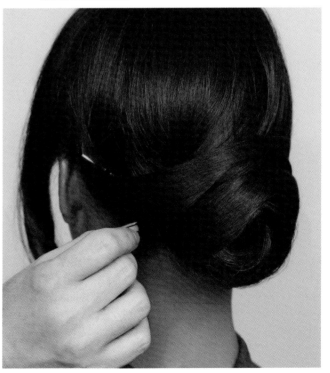

15 Take the remaining back section and cross it over to the right side of the chignon clockwise. Secure with bobby pins. This step can be done using 1 or 2 sections.

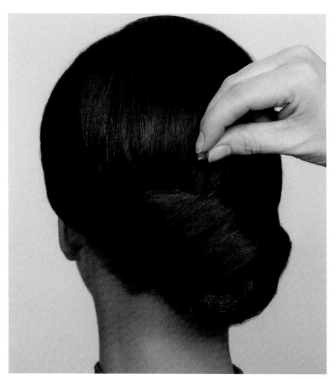

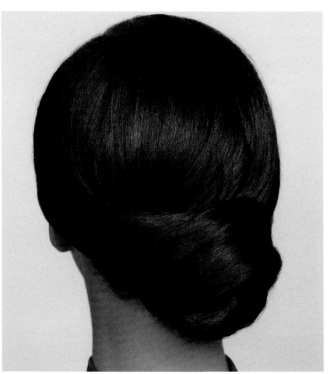

16 Take the left side section and cross it over to the right side of the chignon and secure with bobby pins. Use hairpins to hide any of the bobby pins that are visible.

17 Finish with hair spray.

BUN ON TOP

Bun on Top is a great choice for clients with long hair. Those clients with shorter hair can attach a weft to make the bun larger, so it works for a variety of hair lengths. An added bonus of this hairstyle is that it increases the client's height by 2 to 3 inches!

The hairstyles chosen for this section are Classic Bun on Top, Messy Bun on Top, and Braided Bun on Top.

A filler was used for Classic Bun on Top for fullness, and the front has been teased for volume.

Messy Bun on Top has a filler and wefts attached for height and fullness.

Braided Bun on Top has a braided weft attached for fullness and a braid detail in front.

CLASSIC
BUN ON TOP

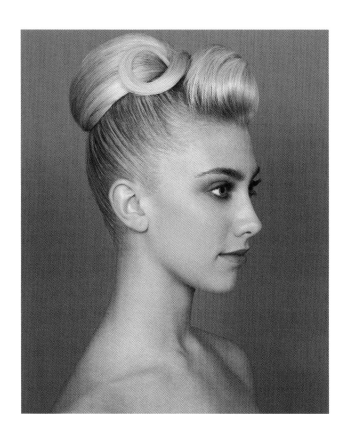 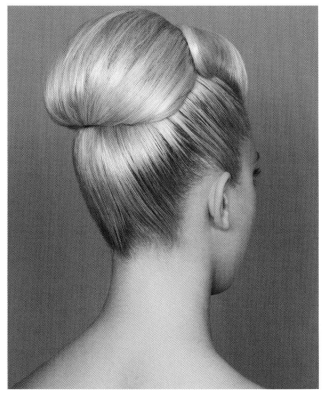

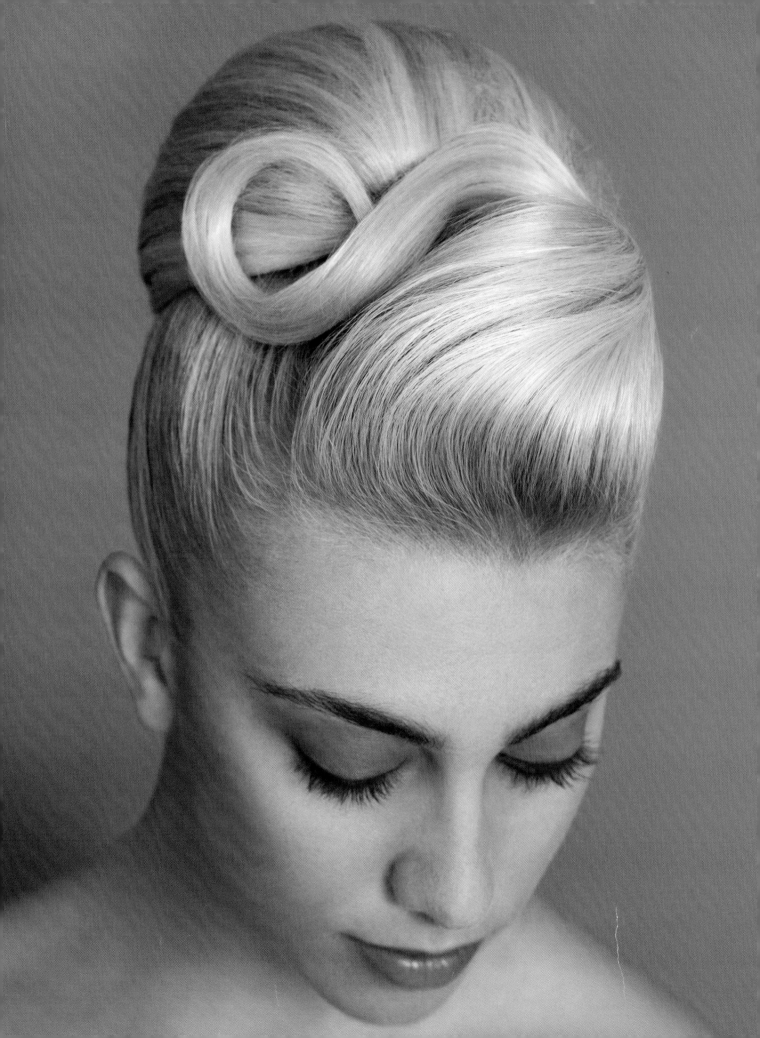

CLASSIC **BUN ON TOP**

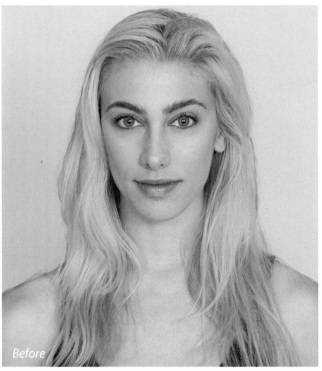

Before

Hair Texture: Fine, straight
Hair Length: Long

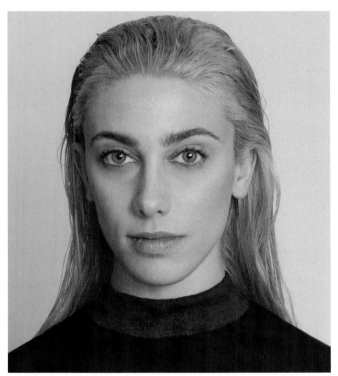

1 Start with hair that has been shampooed and conditioned. Then, apply a styling product to towel-dried hair best suited for the client's hair type and texture.

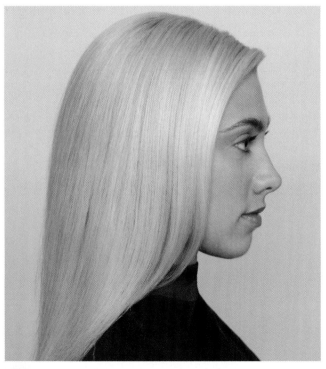

2 Blowdry the hair with a round brush, leaving some body in the hair.

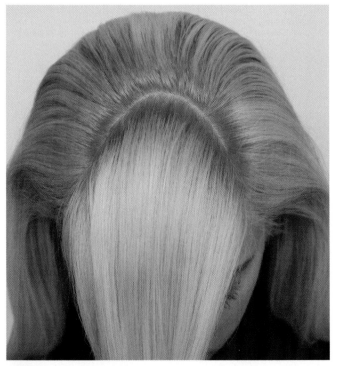

3 Make a U-shaped section in the front from temple to temple extending about 3 inches toward the apex.

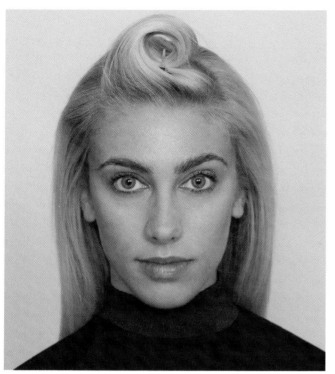

4 Curl the front section and put it in a large pin curl.

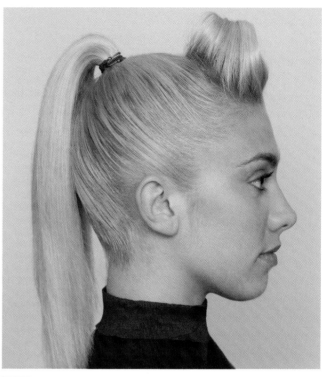

5 Brush the hair up into a high ponytail with a cushion brush, about 1 inch below the apex. Secure with a bungee band.

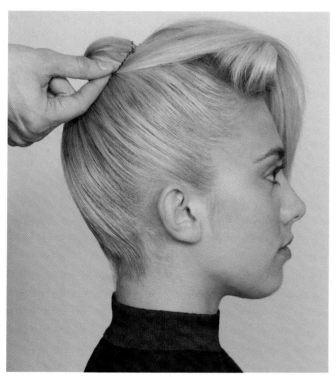

6 Tease the ponytail with a teasing comb. Then, direct the hair above the bungee band and pin with bobby pins.

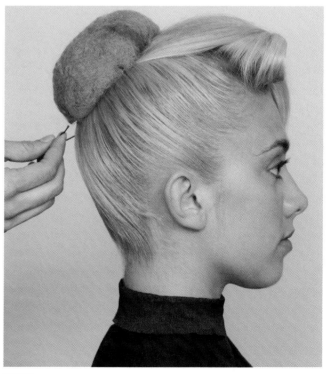

7 Place a filler on top of the ponytail and secure with bobby pins on the outer edge, except the bottom.

Classic Bun on Top   **77**

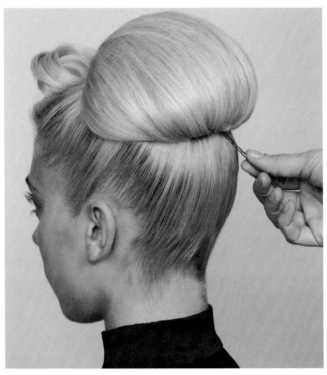

8 Distribute the hair evenly with a cushion brush over the filler while tucking the ends underneath. Pin around the entire outer edge using hairpins.

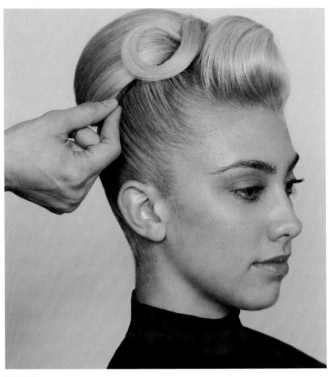

9 Tease the front section and then smooth it. Then, twist the section to the left and place the ends on top of the bun. Secure with hairpins.

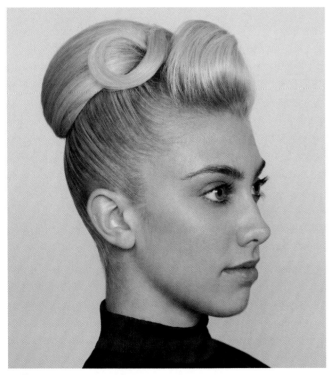

10 Finish with hair spray.

MESSY
BUN ON TOP

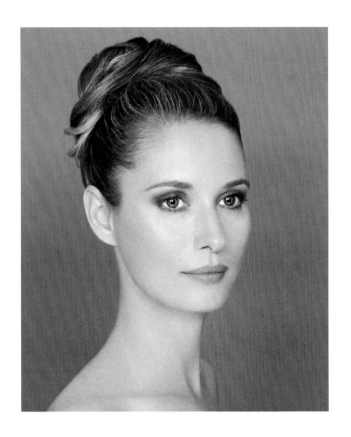 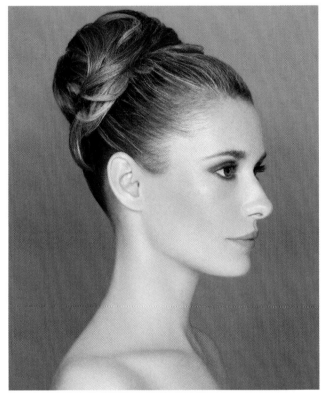

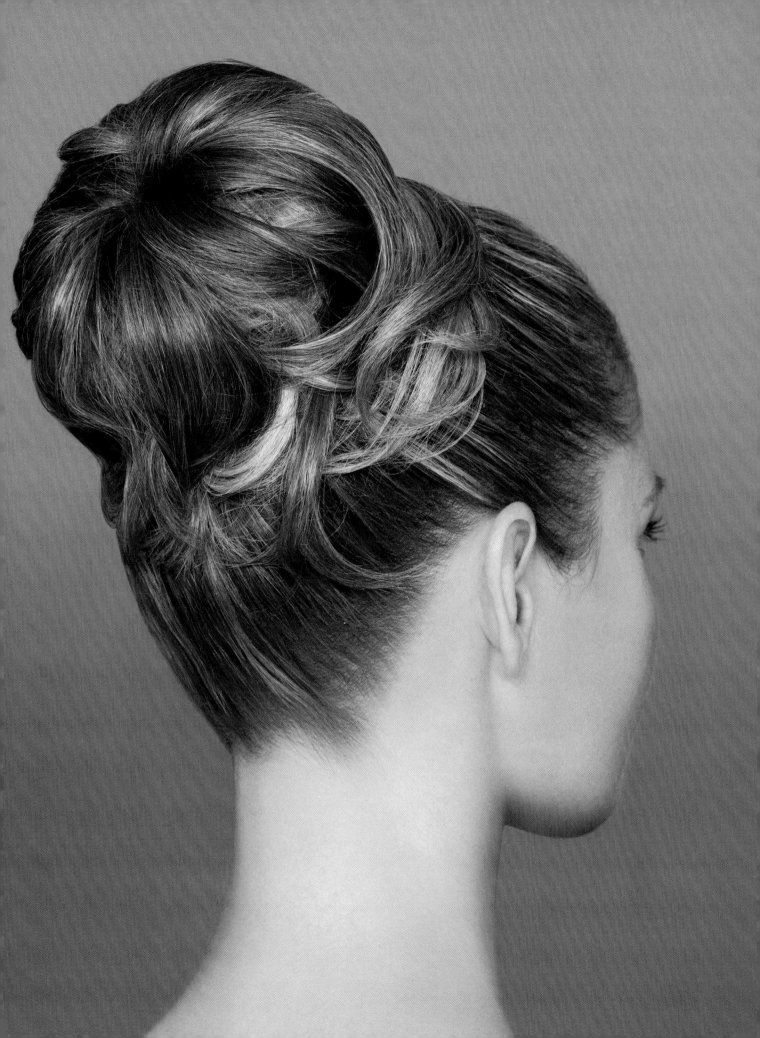

MESSY **BUN ON TOP**

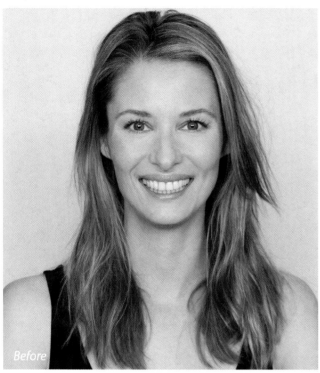

Before

Hair Texture: Straight
Hair Length: Shoulder-length

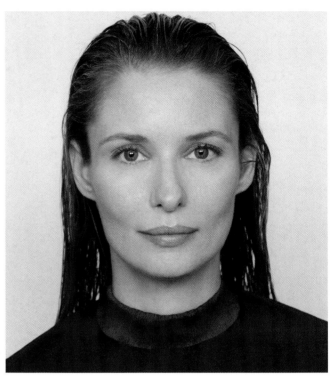

1 Start with hair that has been shampooed and conditioned. Apply a styling product to towel-dried hair best suited for the client's hair type and texture.

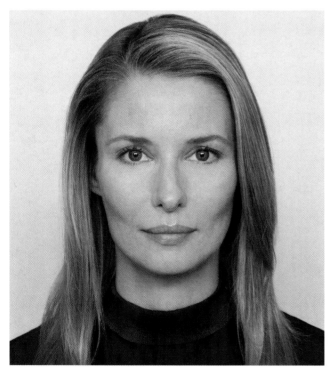

2 Blowdry the client's hair with a round brush, leaving some body in the hair.

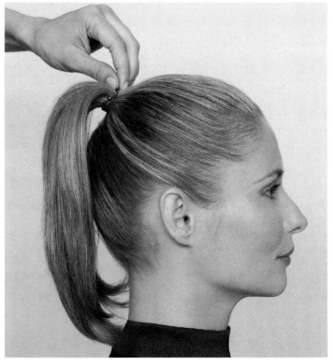

3 Brush the hair up into a high ponytail about 1 inch below the apex. Finger comb the hair to rough it up a bit. Then, secure it with a bungee band.

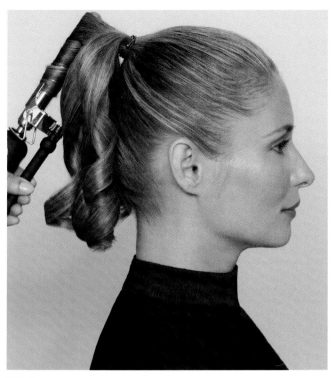

4 Curl the loose hair with a medium-sized curling iron, taking 2-inch sections.

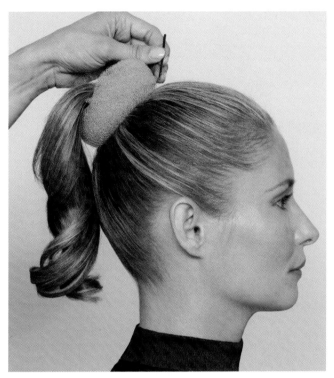

5 Pull the loose hair through a doughnut-shaped filler and secure the filler to the base of the ponytail with bobby pins.

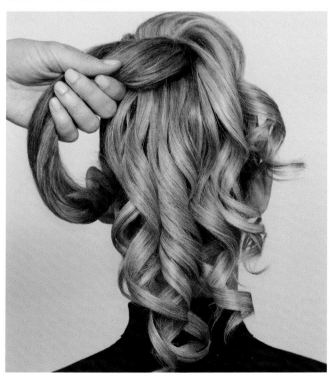

6 Pin a weft of hair around the center of the doughnut-shaped filler. The weft of hair should measure about 6 to 8 inches in length. If it is longer, cut the hair on the weft.

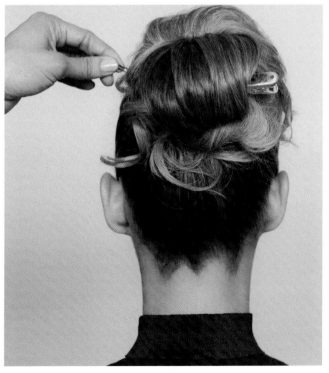

7 Tease the hair on the weft and cover the filler with random pieces of the hair, pinning to the filler. Some of the ends of the hair should be tucked under the filler and some should be left out. It should be a little messy.

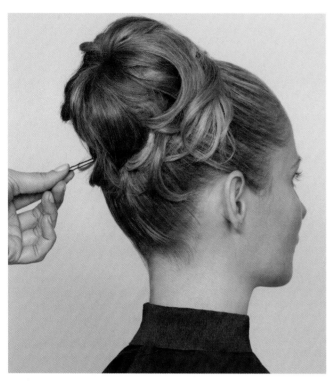

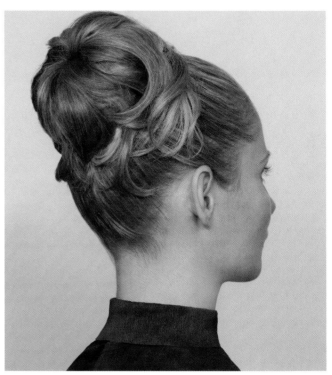

8 Tease the ponytail slightly. Randomly pin about 6 to 8 pieces of the ponytail to the filler and secure with bobby pins. Leave some of the ends out for a tousled look.

9 Finish with texture spray.

BRAIDED
BUN ON TOP

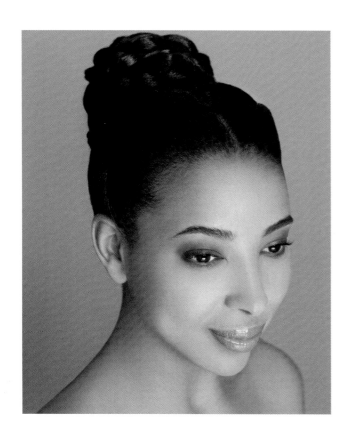
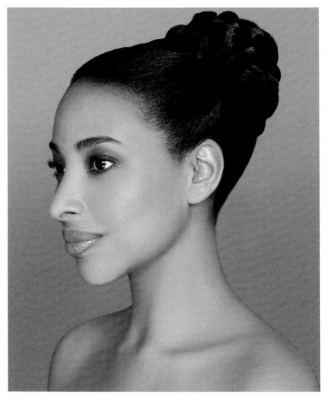

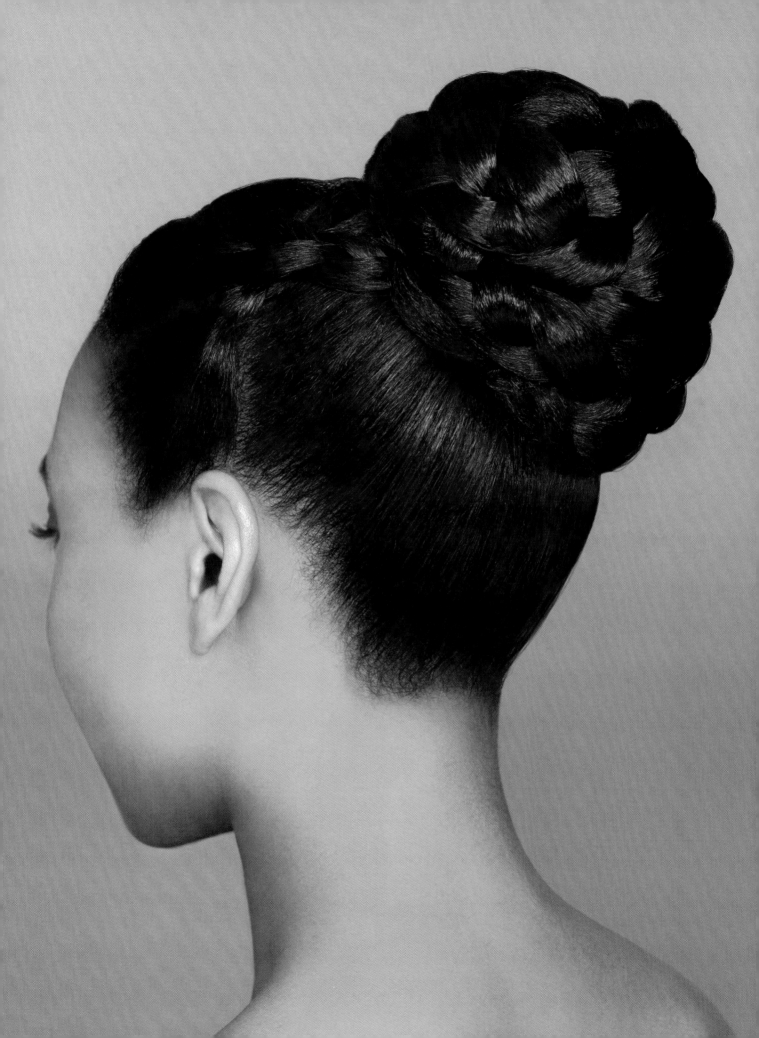

BRAIDED BUN ON TOP

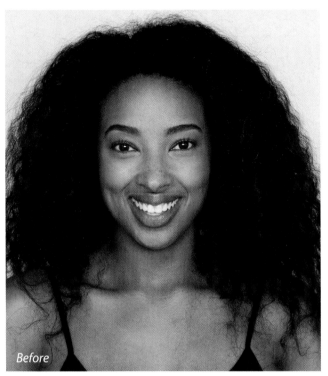

Before

Hair Texture: Thick, curly
Hair Length: Long

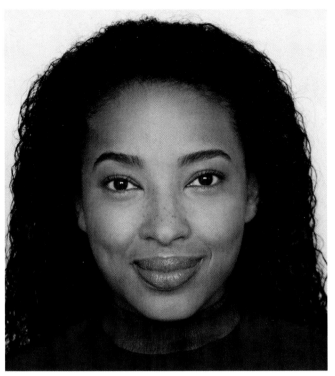

1 Start with hair that has been shampooed and conditioned. Apply a styling product to towel-dried hair best suited for the client's hair type and texture.

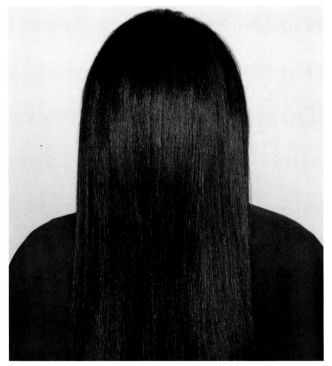

2 Blowdry the hair with a round brush, leaving some body in the hair.

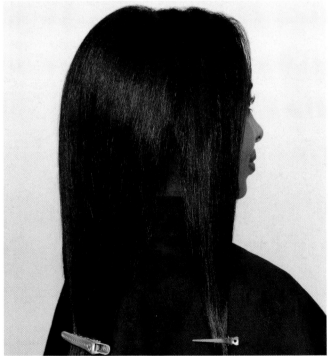

3 Divide the hair from just above the apex to behind the ear. The front should be divided in the center.

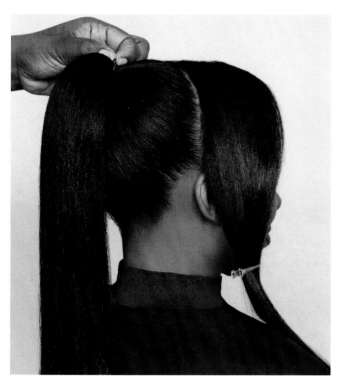

4 Brush the back section of the hair up into a high ponytail about 1 inch below the apex. Then, secure with a bungee band.

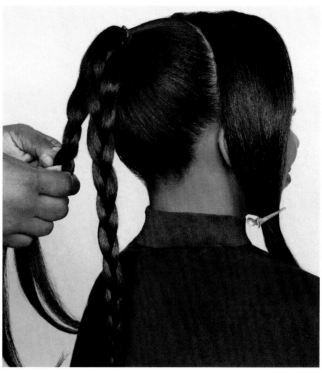

5 Divide the ponytail into 2 pieces and braid each one to the ends.

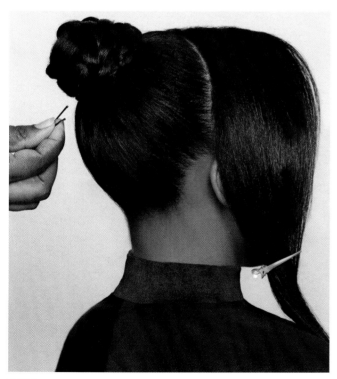

6 Wrap the braids around the bungee band and secure with bobby pins.

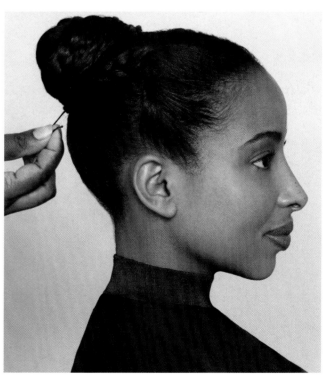

7 Divide the loose hair into 2 sections on each side and braid. Then, crisscross the braids and pin to the bun on each side.

Braided Bun on Top   **89**

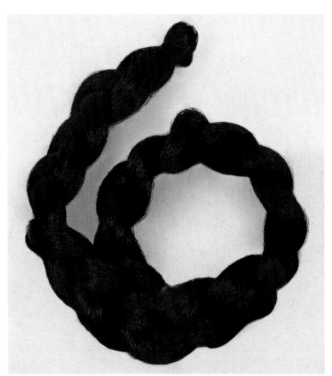

8 Braid a hairpiece about 12 inches in length.

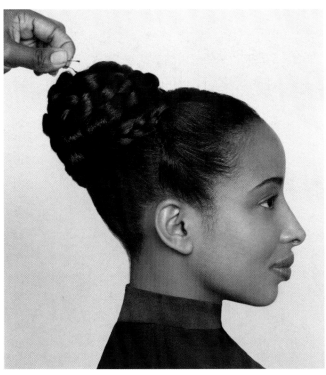

9 Arrange the braided hairpiece randomly on top of the other braids. Then, secure with bobby pins while positioning the braid.

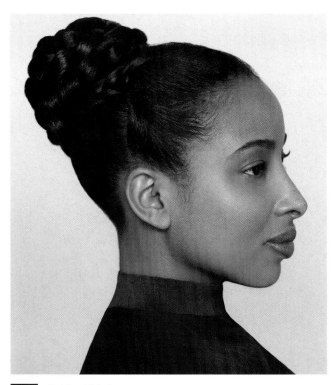

10 Finish with hair spray.

FRENCH
TWIST

Audrey Hepburn's French twist and little black dress captivated audiences in the movie *Breakfast at Tiffany's*. Her hairstyle was emulated around the world and is still being worn today. Her persona epitomizes great style and elegance.

The French twist is achievable with hair a minimum of 6 inches in length. This hairstyle is great for those who do not have long hair but still want to wear their hair up. By adding some volume, teasing, and hair spray, it will stay in place all night. A French twist also can be done on longer hair.

There are four French twist styles in this section: Classic French Twist, Messy French Twist, Low French Twist, and Curly French Twist. We have changed the textures on each French twist to show the versatility of the hairstyle. Also, we have varied the technique to show the different ways in which the style can be achieved.

CLASSIC
FRENCH TWIST

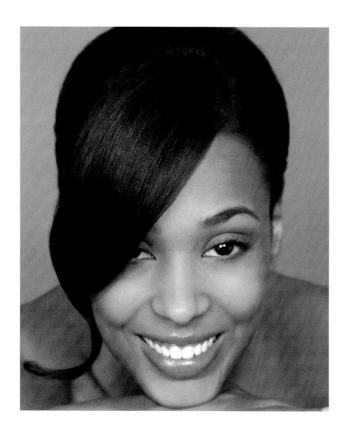
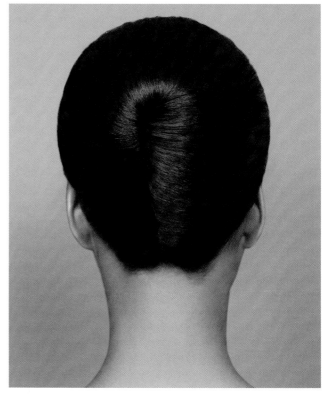

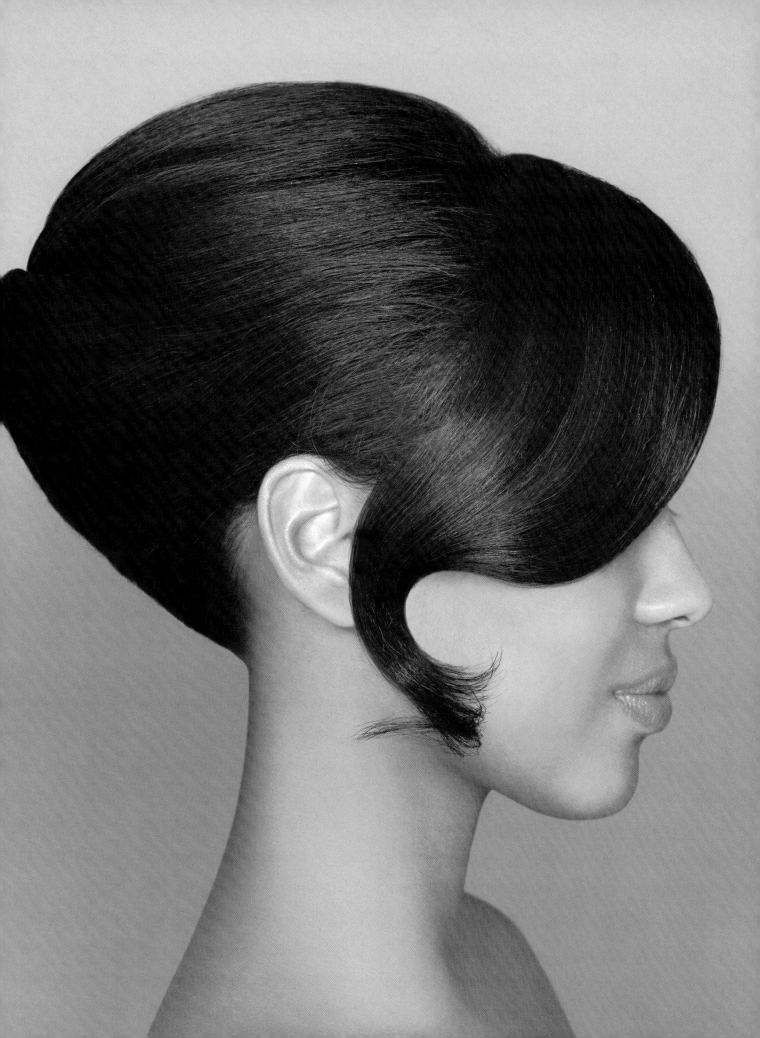

CLASSIC FRENCH TWIST

Before

Hair Texture: Curly
Hair Length: Long

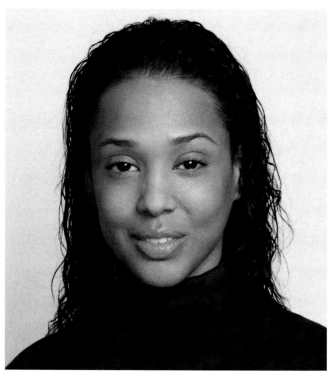

1 Start with hair that has been shampooed and conditioned. Then, apply a styling product best suited for the client's hair type and texture.

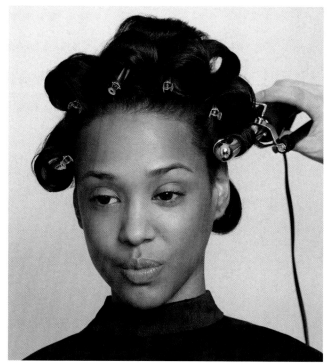

2 Blowdry hair with a round brush and then curl with a medium-sized curling iron. Pin curl each piece as it is curled.

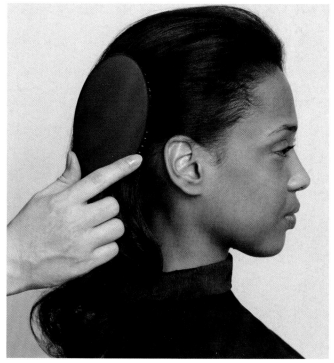

3 Remove the clips and brush the hair thoroughly to remove all the parts.

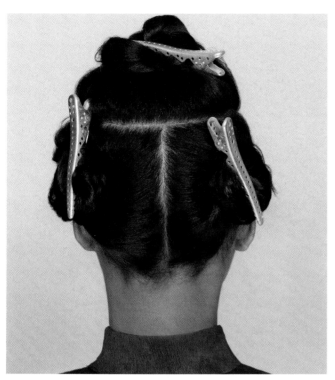

4 Divide the hair into 3 sections. The crown section goes from temple to temple and stops 2 inches below the apex. The last 2 sections are from the middle of the back combined with the hair on the sides.

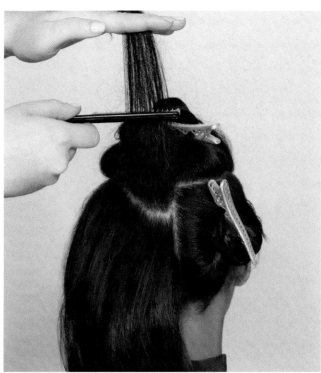

5 Tease the left section.

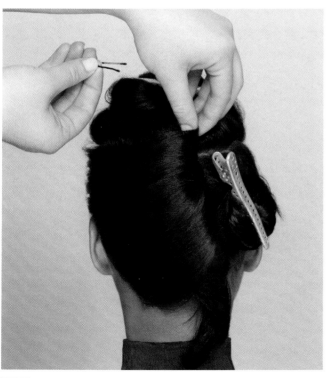

6 Smooth the teased left section with a cushion brush and direct it toward the center of the back. Then, make a loop with the hair at the top of the section and turn it toward the center.

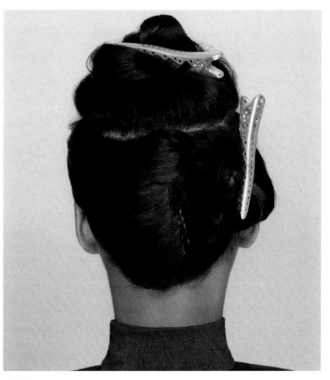

7 Tuck the ends of the hair inside the opening where the hair overlaps. Pin with bobby pins in a row on top of the hair to secure.

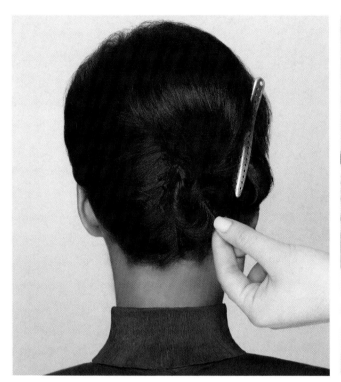

8 Part the hair on the side. Then tease the top section and smooth it back with a cushion brush. Make sure to blend the top hair with the sides. Pin the top section along the crease and secure with bobby pins.

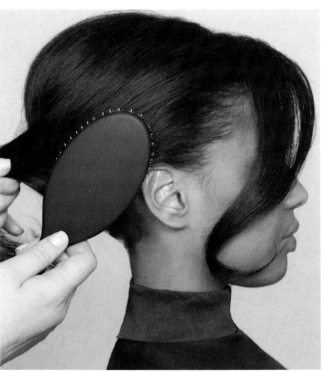

9 Tease the right section, smooth, and direct toward the center.

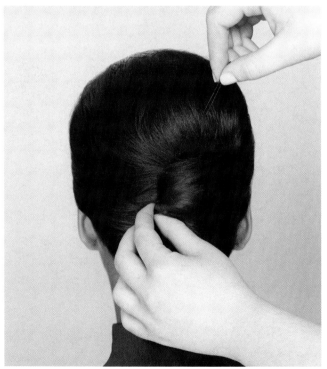

10 Make a loop at the top of the section and pin with hairpins in the crease to conceal. Starting from the bottom, make a neat fold and pin with hairpins.

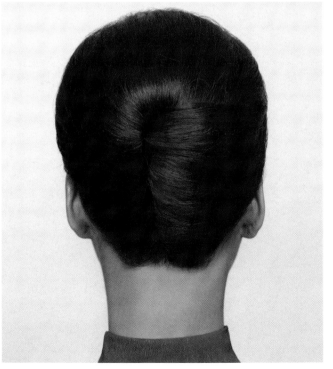

11 Finish with hair spray.

LOW
FRENCH TWIST

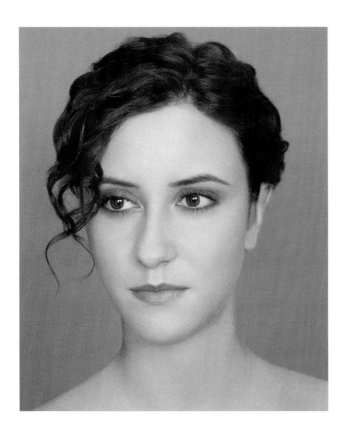
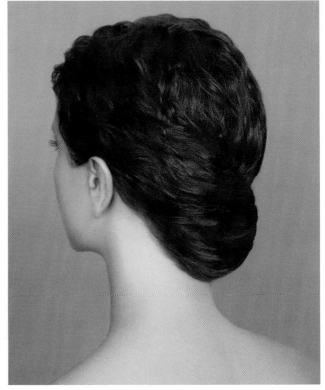

All photos Copyright © 2015 Milady, a part of Cengage Learning®. Photography by Timothy C. Johnson.

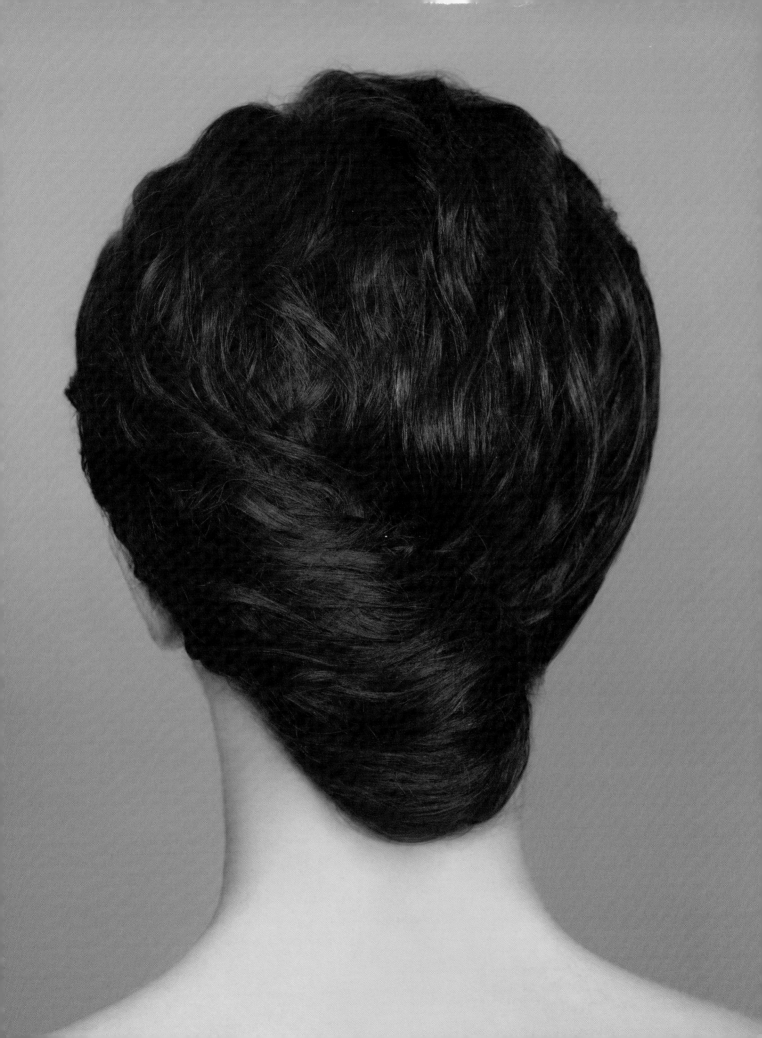

LOW **FRENCH TWIST**

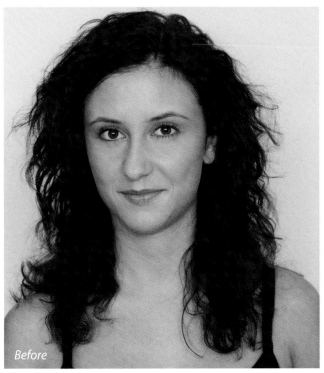

Before

Hair Texture: Curly
Hair Length: Shoulder-length

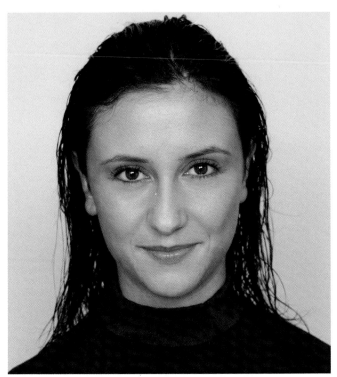

1 Start with hair that has been shampooed and conditioned. Then, apply a styling product best suited for the client's hair type and texture.

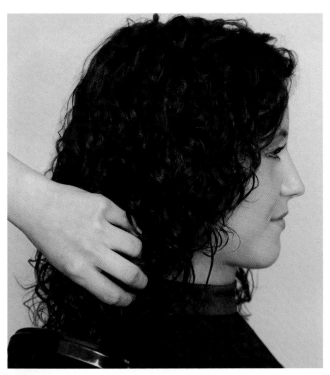

2 Dry naturally curly hair with a diffuser.

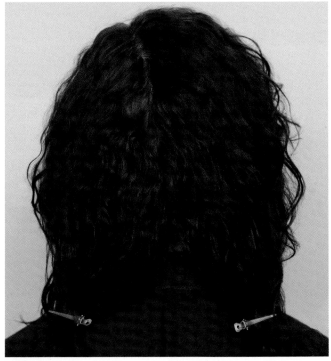

3 Establish a side part on the left side. Then, divide the hair into 2 sections, from the side part toward the middle of the back.

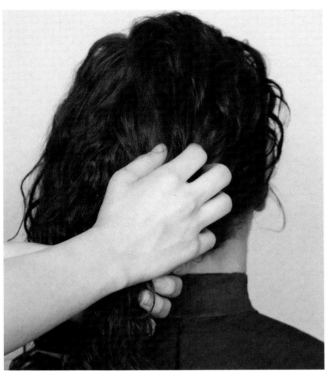

4 Starting with the right side, use your fingers to direct the hair toward the back center.

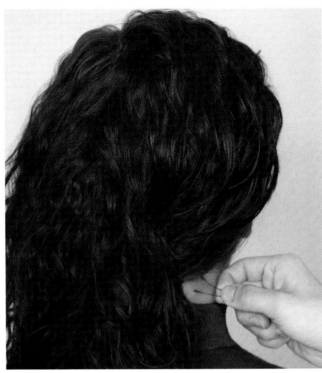

5 Pin the hair flat to the head with bobby pins at an angle. The height of the pins should be about 3 inches.

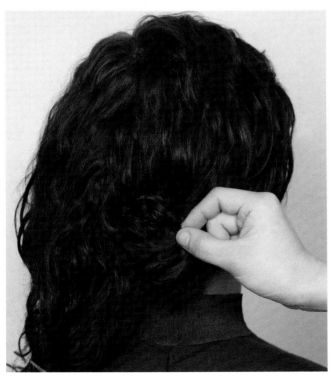

6 Make a flat pin curl with the loose hair and pin to the head. Crisscross the pins to secure.

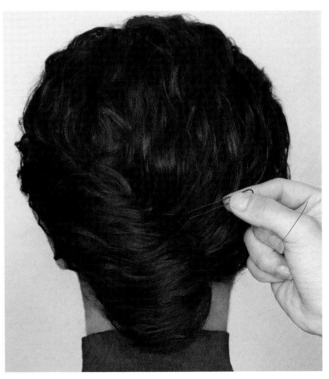

7 Direct the left side past the center using your fingers. Make a loop over the pins and secure the hair in the fold with hair pins. Then, tuck the ends inside and pin from the bottom.

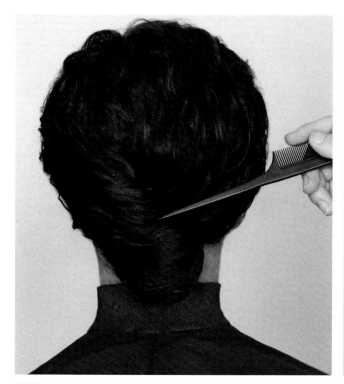

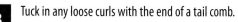

8 Tuck in any loose curls with the end of a tail comb.

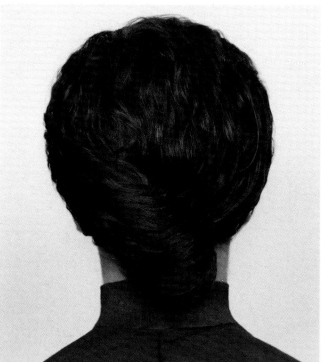

9 Finish with texture spray.

MESSY
FRENCH TWIST

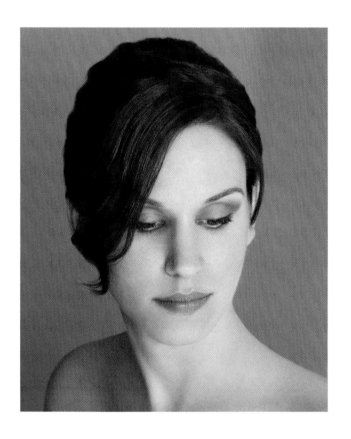
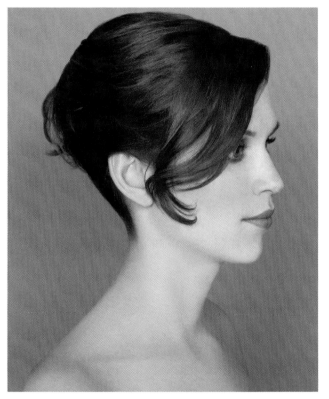

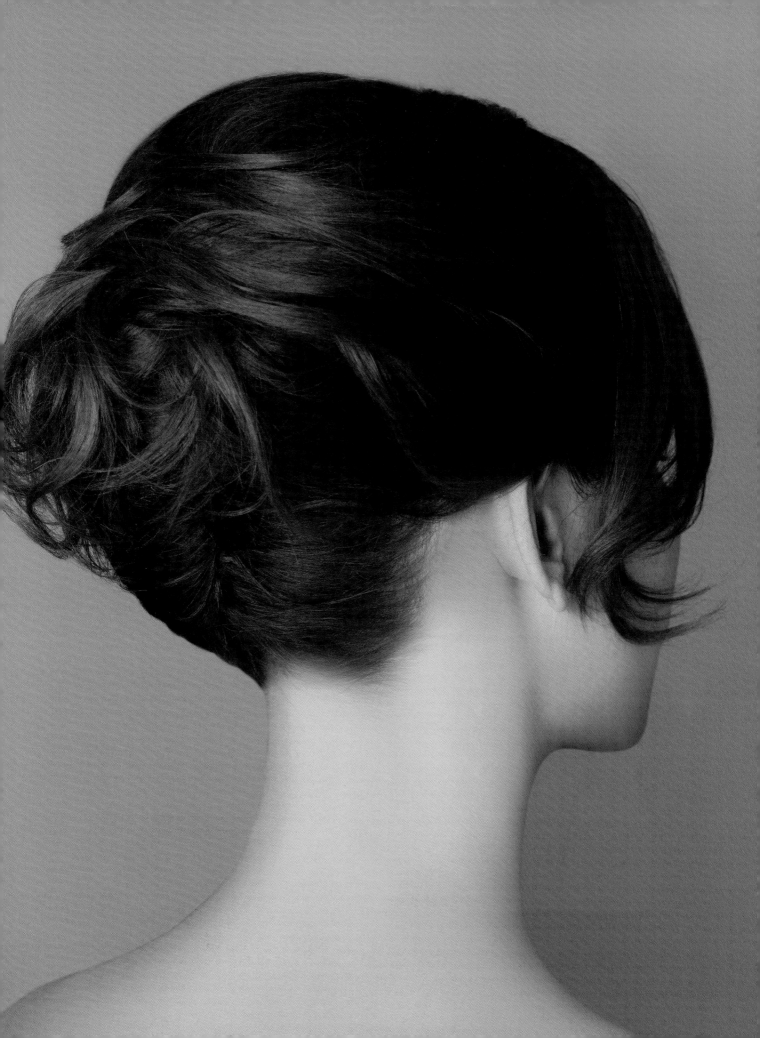

MESSY FRENCH TWIST

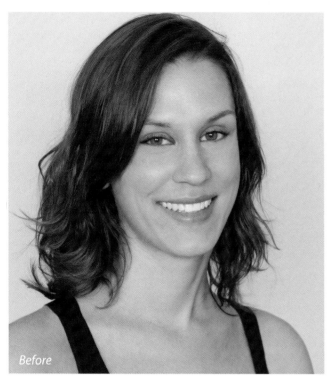

Before

Hair Texture: Fine, straight
Hair Length: Above the shoulders

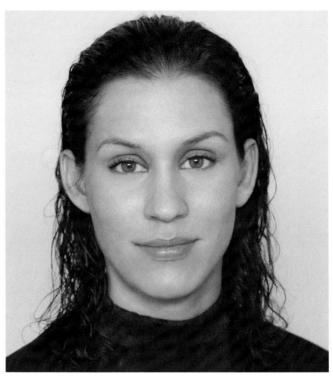

1 Start with hair that has been shampooed and conditioned. Then, apply a styling product best suited for the client's hair type and texture.

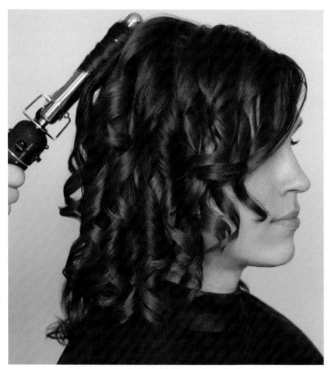

2 Blowdry the hair with a round brush. Then, curl the hair with a medium-sized curling iron.

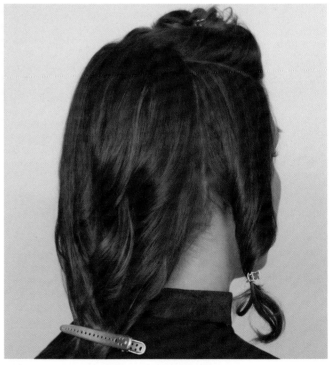

3 Divide the hair into 4 sections. The back section is divided from behind the apex and ears. The side sections are divided at the temples, and the top section is the fourth section.

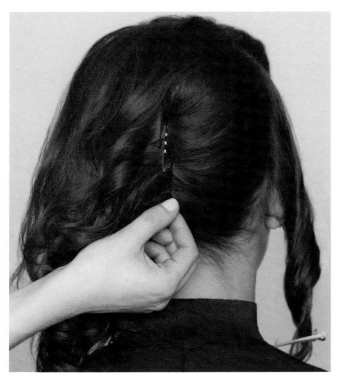

4 Tease the back section and smooth with a cushion brush. Next, use your fingers to direct the hair to the left side and place bobby pins up the center.

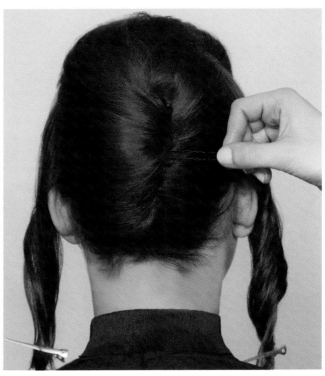

5 Fold the left side over the right side while tucking the ends inside to make a roll. Pin in the crease with hairpins from the bottom up.

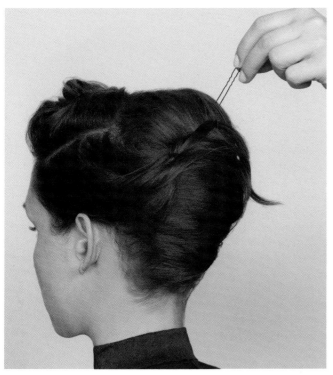

6 Divide the left side in 2 subsections. The first subsection is pinned to the back while leaving the ends out. The second subsection is also pinned to the back. Be sure not to pull the sides too tight.

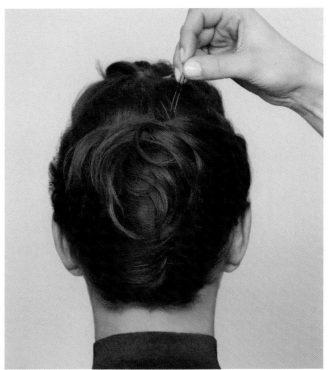

7 Repeat step 6 on the right side.

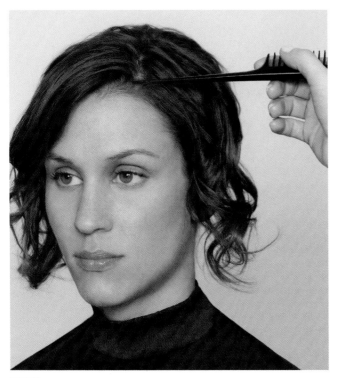

8 Establish a side zigzag part with the end of the tail comb and separate a few pieces around the face for softness.

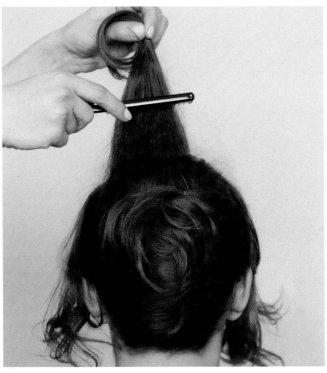

9 Tease the top section. Then, divide it into 3 subsections and pin these to the back with hairpins, leaving some of the ends out.

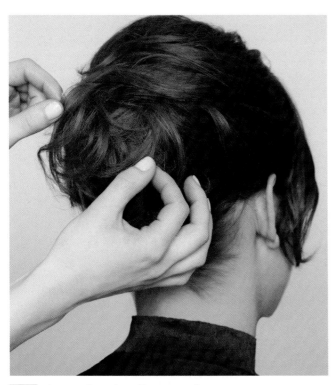

10 Arrange the ends and hairpins in place.

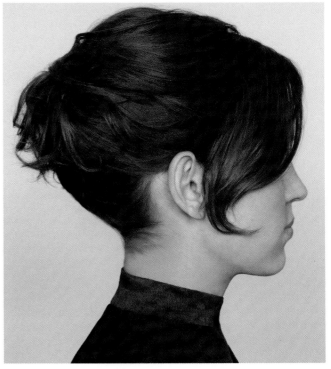

11 Finish with texture spray.

CURLY
FRENCH TWIST

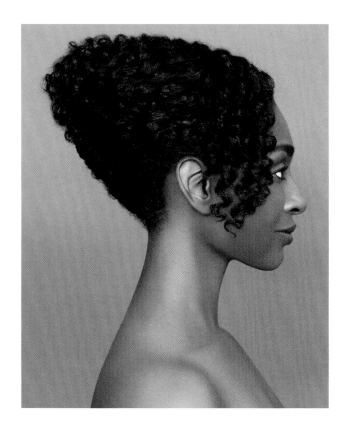
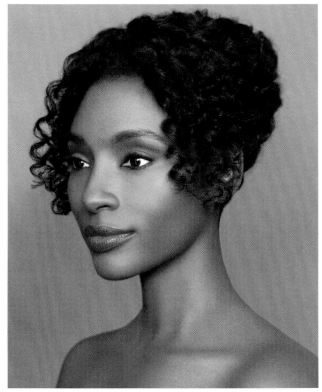

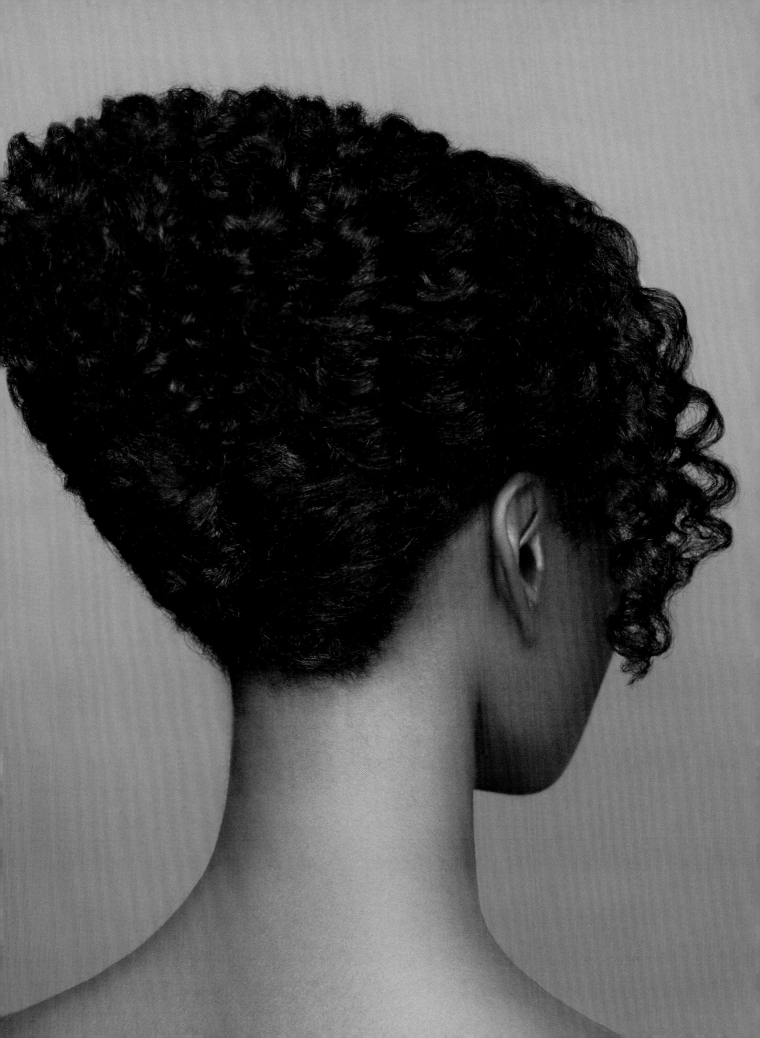

CURLY FRENCH TWIST

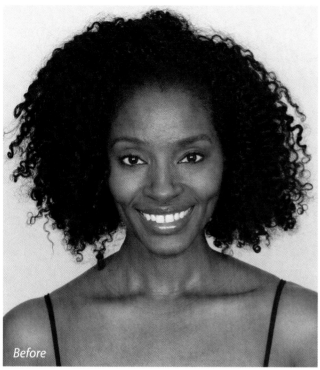

Before

Hair Texture: Curly
Hair Length: Shoulder-length

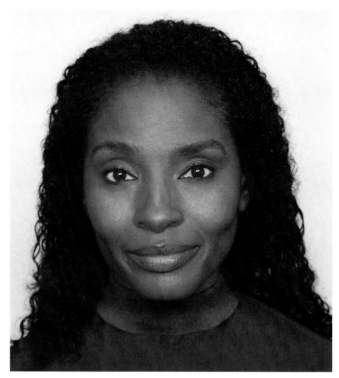

1 Start with hair that has been shampooed and conditioned. Then, apply a styling product best suited for the client's hair type and texture.

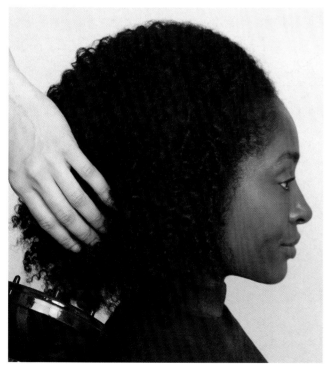

2 Dry the hair with a diffuser.

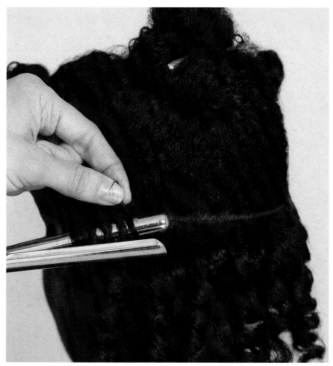

3 Curl the hair by wrapping 1-inch sections around a small curling iron.

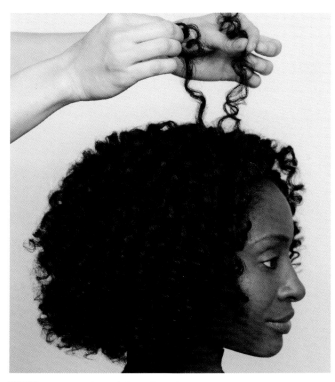

4 Separate the curls by pulling them apart.

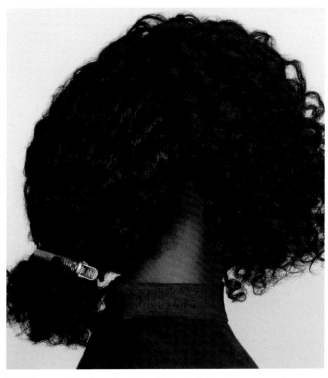

5 Divide the front hair from the back, behind the apex and ears. Then, divide the hair down the center in the front.

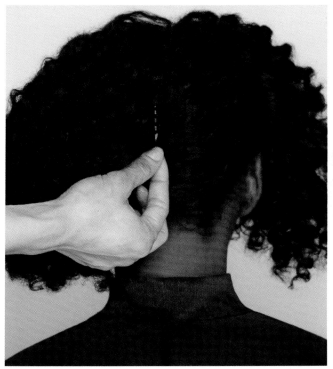

6 Starting with the back section, direct the hair to the left side and pin with bobby pins up the center.

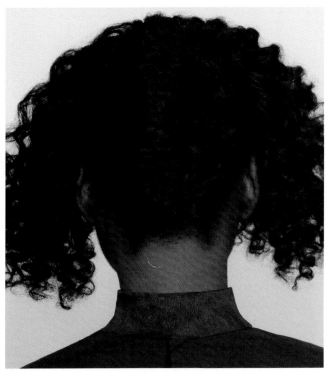

7 Loop the left back section over the right side and pin in the crease with hairpins from the bottom to the top.

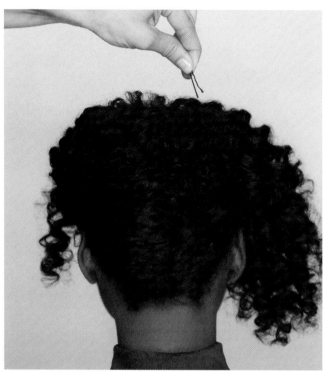

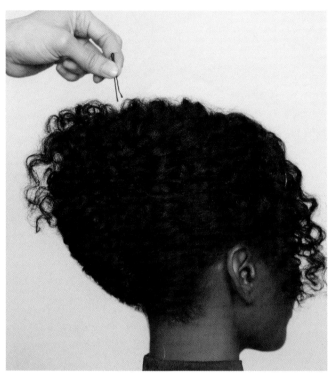

8 Divide the left side section into 2 or 3 subsections. Then, loosely pin each subsection to the top of the roll in back and secure with bobby pins. Leave hair around the face.

9 Repeat step 8 on the right side.

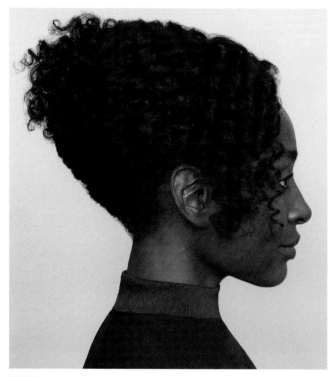

10 Finish with texture spray.

FAUX BOB

The faux bob is not a traditional updo because in this style, long hair is transformed into what appears to be a bob haircut. It is a great illusion—everyone will think the client has cut her hair. Whether curly, wavy, or straight, the faux bob is perfect for all hair textures.

The following faux bobs have been chosen for this section: Classic Faux Bob, Faux Bob with Braid, and Asymmetrical Faux Bob.

A cylinder-shaped filler is used to support the construction of the Classic Faux Bob, and soft pieces are left around the face to create an effortless look.

Faux Bob with a Braid has been looped on top of the hair to show variety in technique, and the braid is intertwined as an added detail.

Asymmetrical Faux Bob has a cylinder-shaped filler to aid in the construction. It also has a piece of hair draped over the back as an added detail.

CLASSIC
FAUX BOB

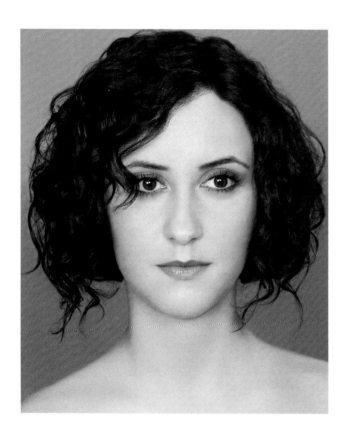
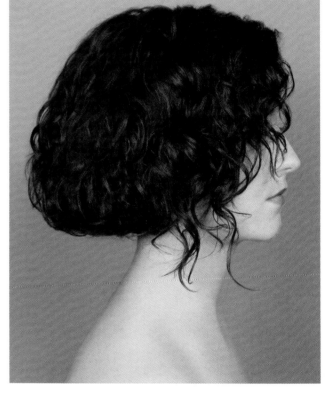

All photos Copyright © 2015 Milady, a part of Cengage Learning®. Photography by Timothy C. Johnson.

120 Classic Faux Bob

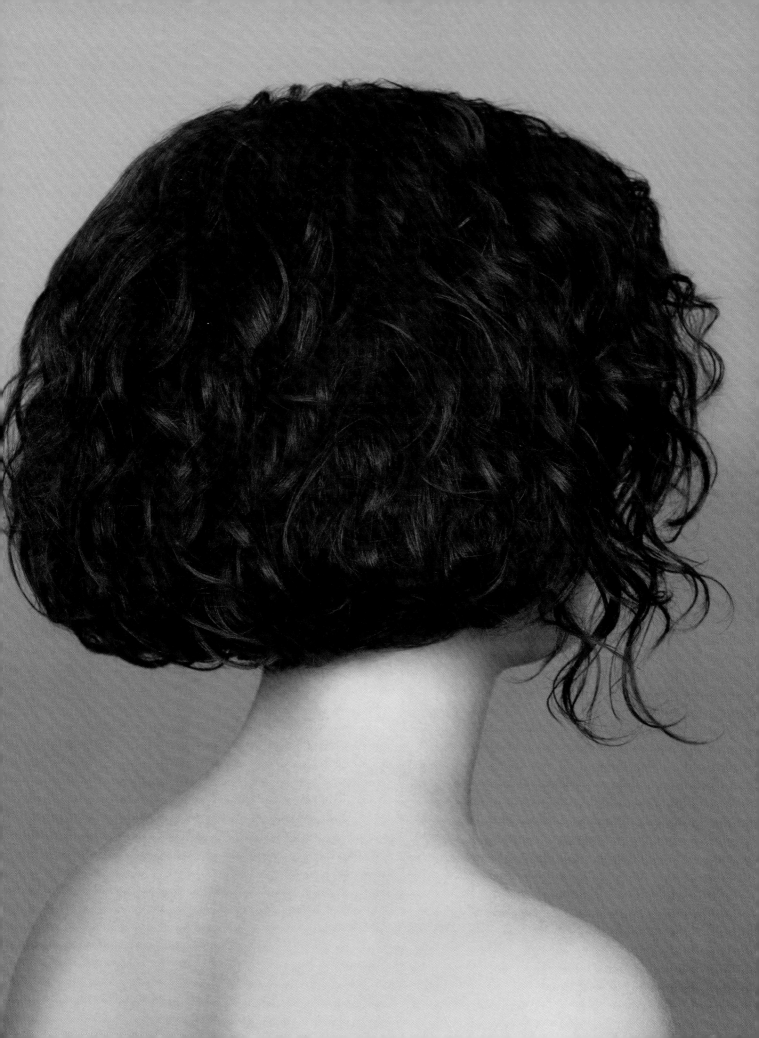

CLASSIC **FAUX BOB**

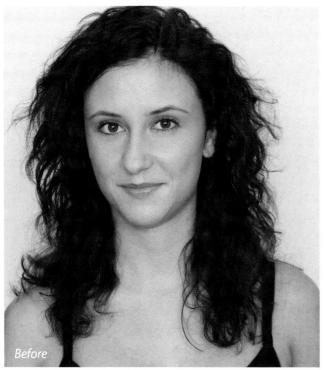

Before

Hair Texture: Curly
Hair Length: Shoulder-length

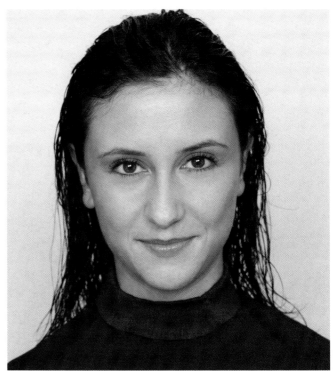

1 Start with hair that has been shampooed and conditioned. Then, apply a styling product to towel-dried hair best suited for the client's hair type and texture.

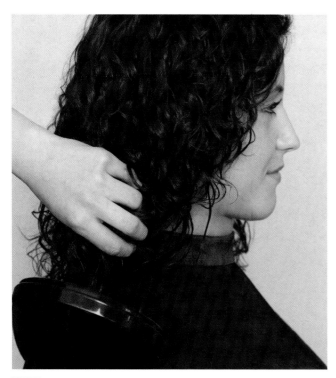

2 Dry naturally curly hair with a diffuser.

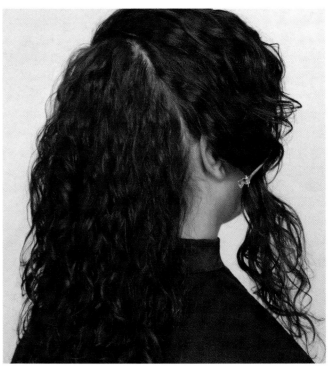

3 Establish a side part. Then, section the hair from behind the apex to just behind the ears.

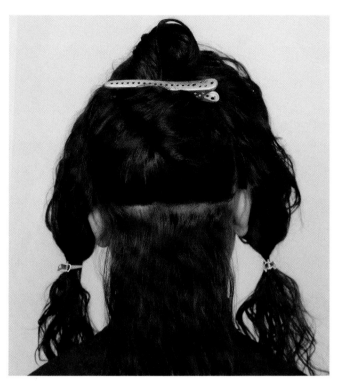

4 Divide the back section horizontally about 2 inches above the hairline. Clip the rest of the section up.

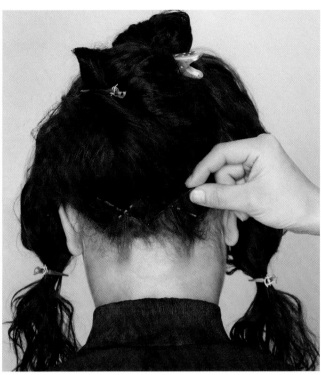

5 Tease the back section. Then, lift the section straight up and place a row of crisscrossed bobby pins.

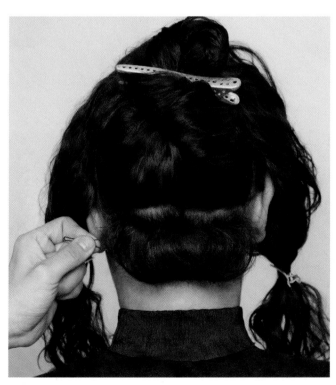

6 Loop the ends of the hair under and pin into the row of pins.

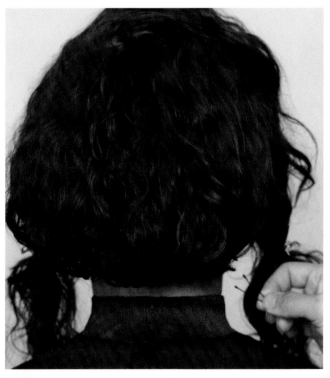

7 Take another 2-inch horizontal section, tease it, and split it into 2 subsections. Then, loop the ends of each subsection under and pin into the row of pins. Repeat for the last back section.

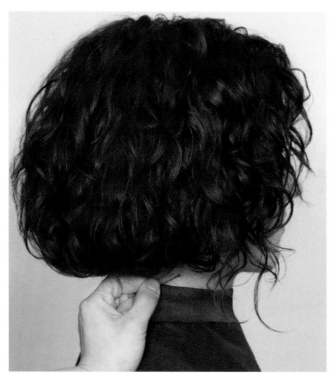

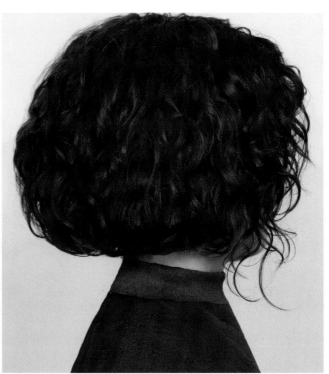

8   Leave some hair around the face. Loop each of the side sections under and pin to the back section, securing with bobby pins.

9   Finish with hair spray.

FAUX
BOB WITH A BRAID

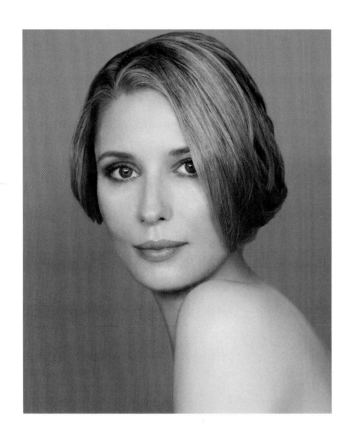
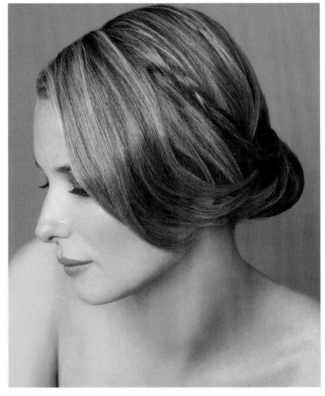

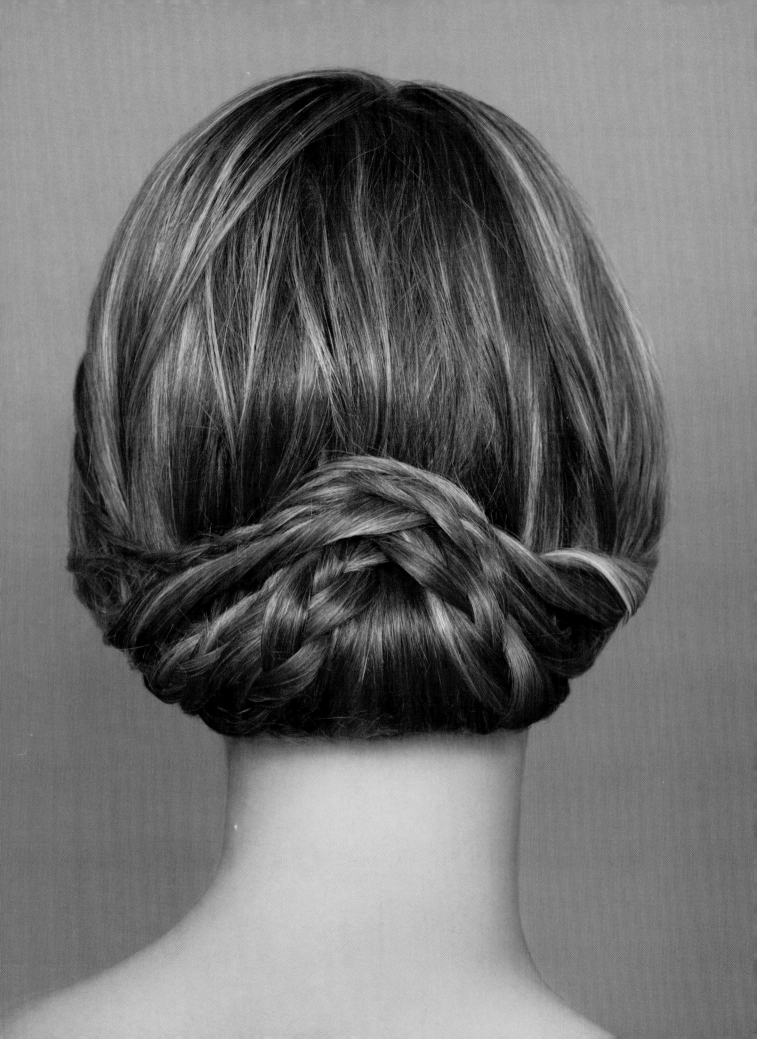

FAUX BOB WITH A BRAID

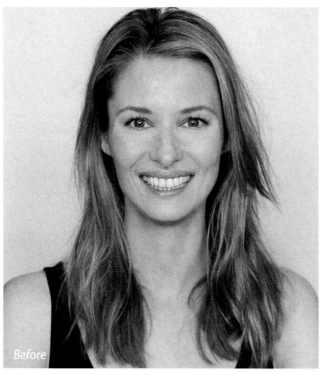

Before

Hair Texture: Straight
Hair Length: Shoulder-length

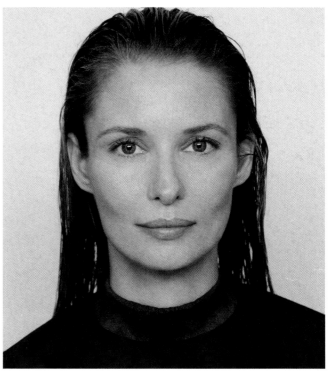

1 Start with hair that has been shampooed and conditioned. Then, apply a styling product to towel-dried hair best suited for the client's hair type and texture.

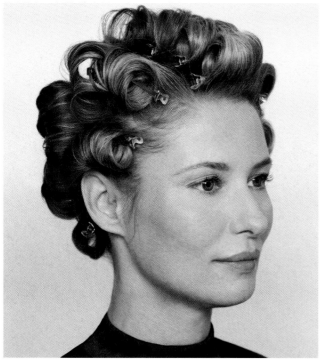

2 Blowdry the hair with a round brush, leaving lots of body in the hair. Establish a side part and then curl the hair with a medium-sized curling iron. Clip each piece as it is curled.

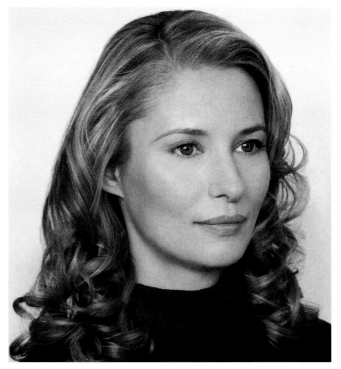

3 Open the curls with your fingers.

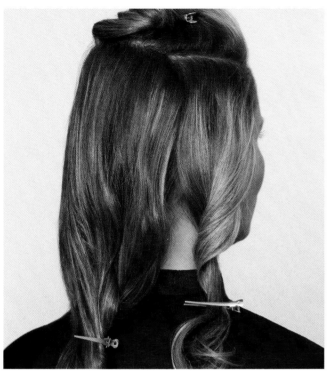

4 Section the hair from behind the apex to just behind the ears.

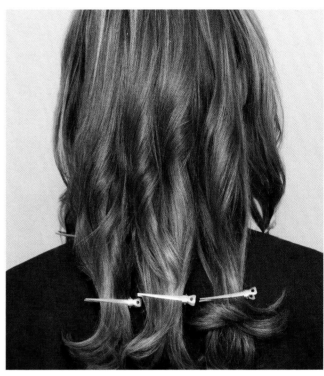

5 Divide the back section into 3 vertical sections.

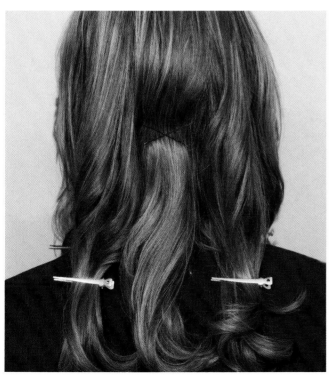

6 Tease the center section slightly. Then, pin on top of the center section with crisscrossed bobby pins.

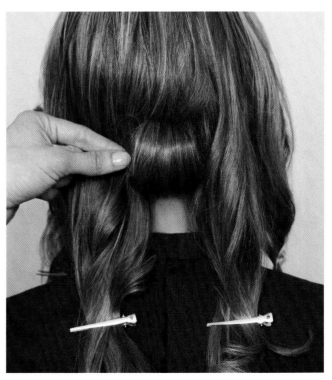

7 Loop the hair upward and secure with bobby pins.

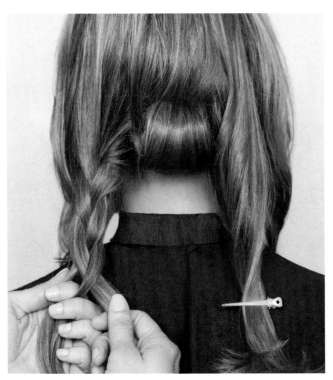

8 Make a loose braid with the left subsection about 2 inches away from the scalp.

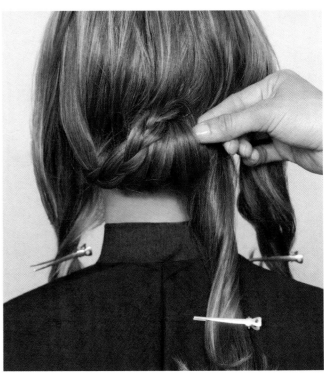

9 Drape the braid over the previous section and secure. Make sure to tuck in the ends of the braid.

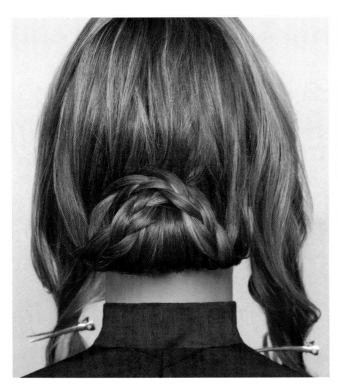

10 Repeat steps 8 and 9 on the left back section.

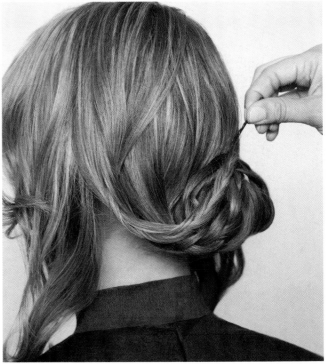

11 Divide the side section into 2 subsections. Braid the subsection near the ear about 3 inches from the scalp, then drape it over the back section and secure.

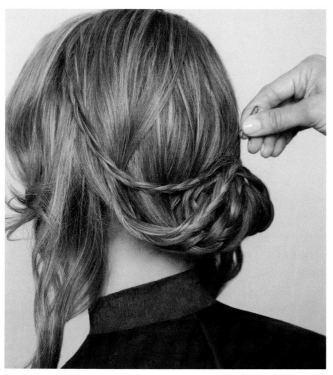

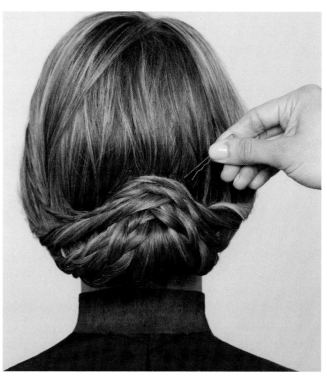

12 Make a loose braid about 1 inch from the hairline and scalp and pin it to the back, using hairpins to secure.

13 Twist the last side subsection and drape it over the back section, securing it with bobby pins and hairpins. Then repeat steps 11, 12, and 13 on the right side section.

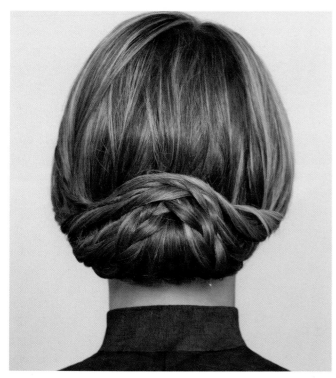

14 Finish with texture spray.

ASSYMETRICAL
FAUX BOB

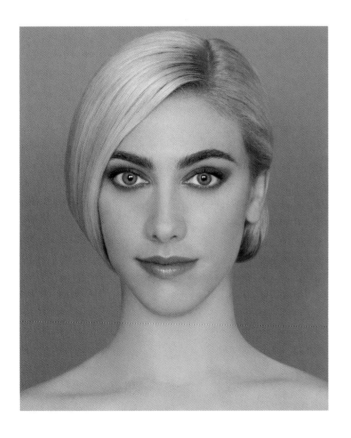 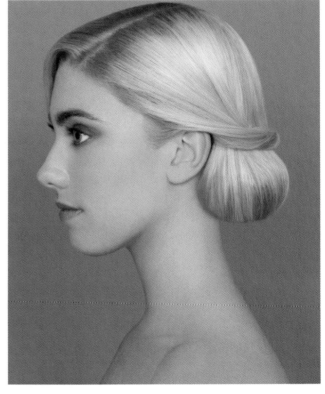

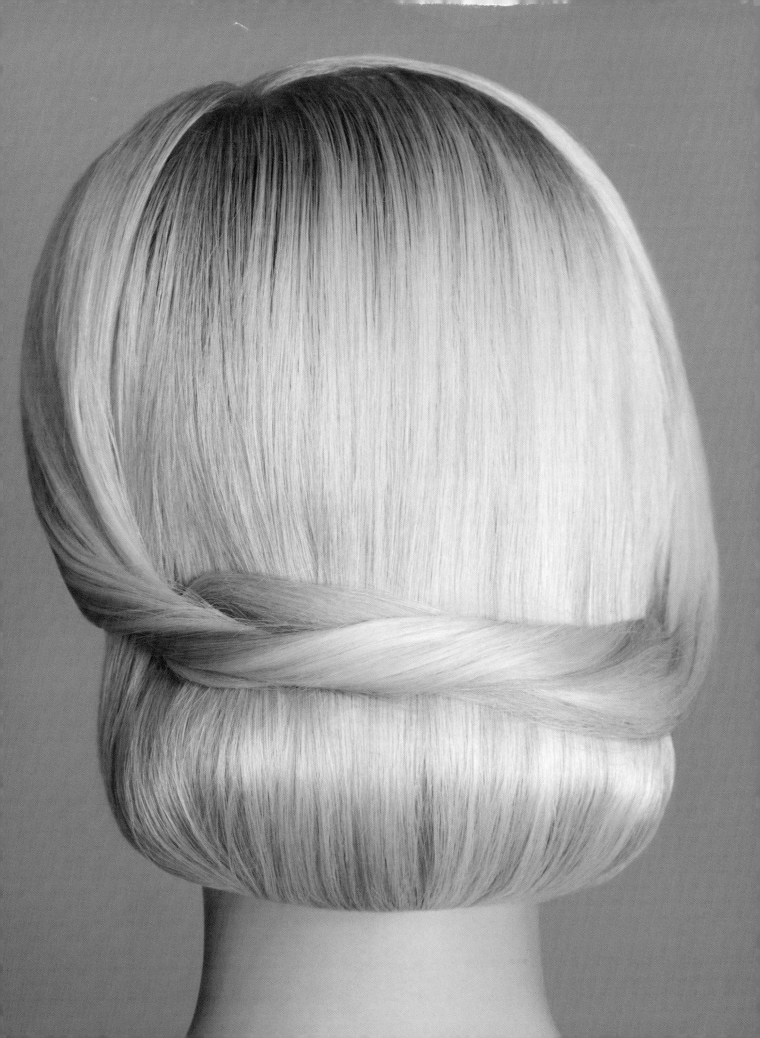

ASSYMETRICAL FAUX BOB

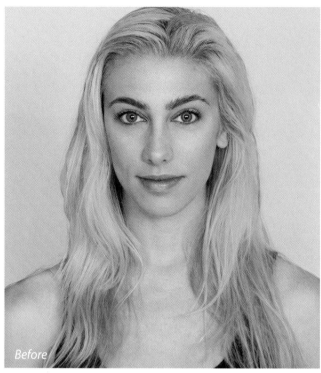

Before

Hair Texture: Fine, straight
Hair Length: Long

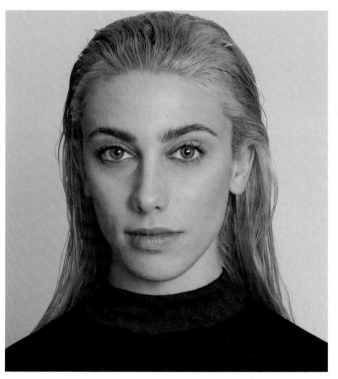

1 Start with hair that has been shampooed and conditioned. Then, apply a styling product to towel-dried hair best suited for the client's hair type and texture.

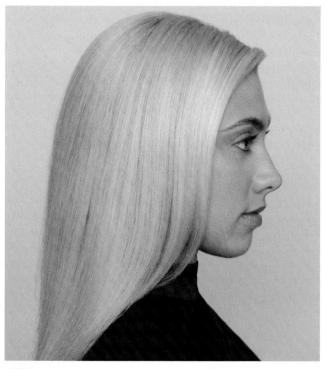

2 Blowdry hair with a round brush, leaving body in the hair.

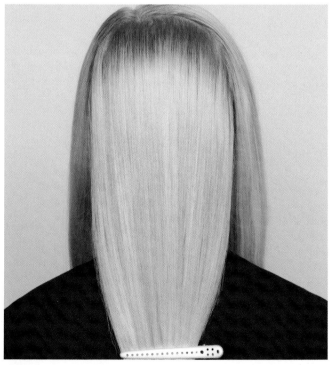

3 Establish a side part. Then, section the hair from behind the apex to just behind the ears.

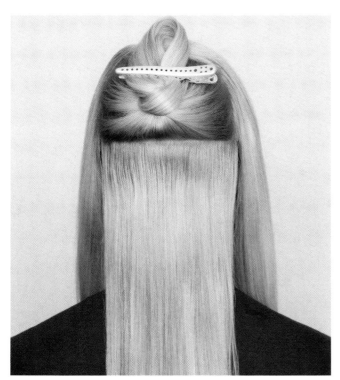

4 Horizontally divide the back section in half.

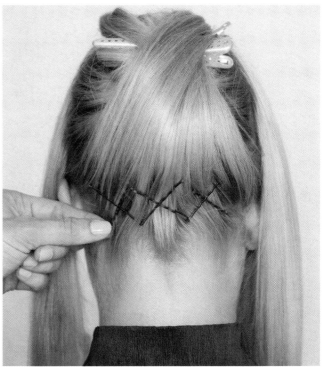

5 Tease the back subsection. Then lift the section up and place a crisscrossed row of bobby pins.

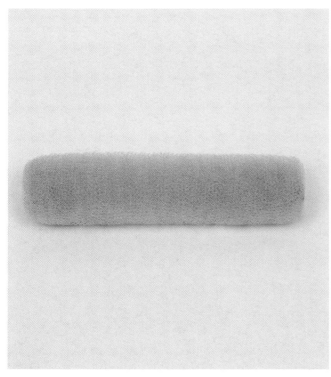

6A Use a tube-shaped filler.

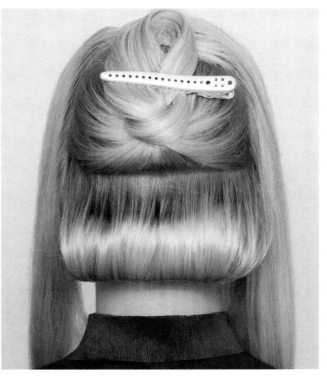

6B Subdivide the back section horizontally about 2 1/2 inches from the hairline. Then, roll the section on the filler and secure with bobby pins. The roll should be positioned at the hairline.

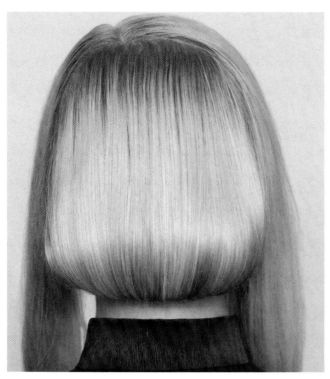

7 Use the rest of the back section to cover the previous section. Secure underneath with bobby pins.

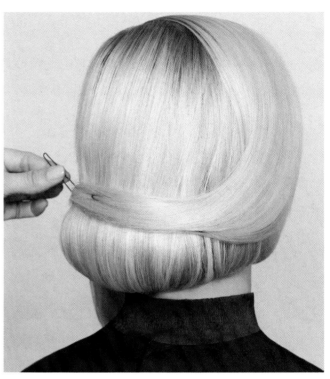

8 Pin the right side back on top of the back section to the far left. Secure with hairpins.

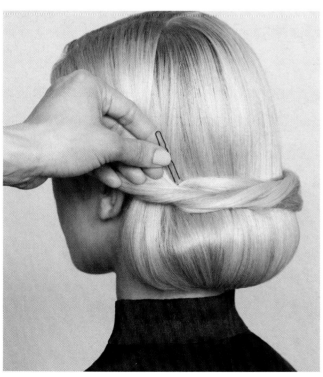

9 Divide the left section into 1 or 2 subsections. Twist the subsection(s) slightly and drape over the back section. Secure with hairpins.

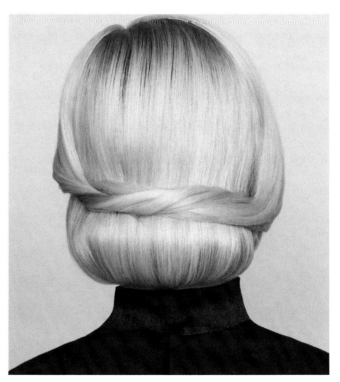

10 Finish with hair spray.

UP IN PIECES

Up in Pieces is a great option for clients who want a loose, soft updo. Because these hairstyles are constructed piece by piece, the technique provides you with a lot of control over how tight and tousled you make the hairstyle. Leaving some pieces sticking out softens the look further and gives the hairstyle an effortless feel.

The hairstyles chosen for this section are Low in Pieces, Fallen Pieces, and Curly Pieces. A small filler is attached to Curly Pieces for added fullness. When an updo is constructed piece by piece, it separates the hair and gives it a done-but-undone look. These hairstyles are great options for women with hair a minimum of 6 inches in length and can also be done on longer hair.

LOW
IN PIECES

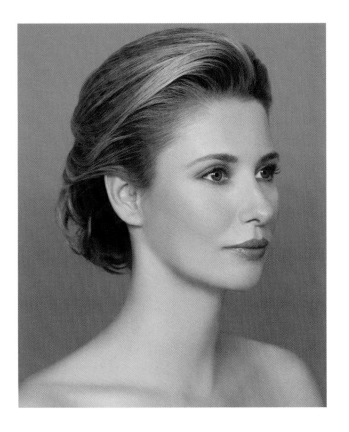
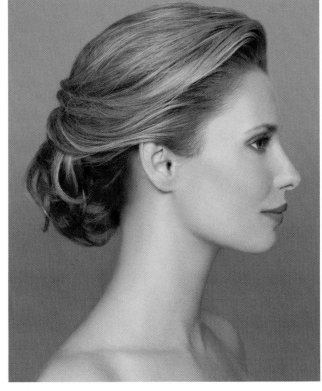

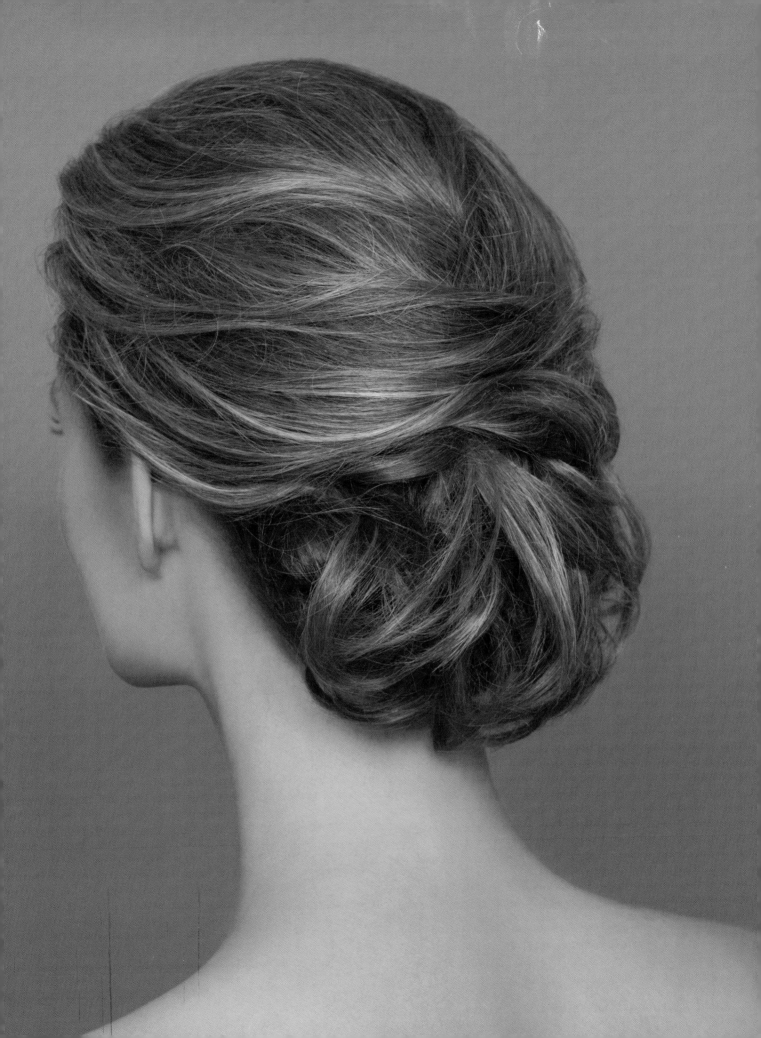

LOW **IN PIECES**

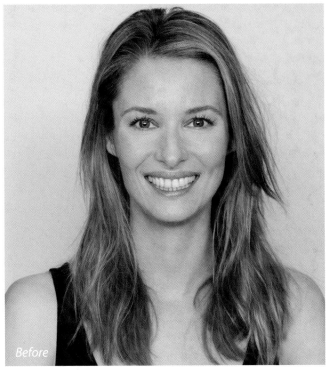

Before

Hair Texture: Straight
Hair Length: Shoulder-length

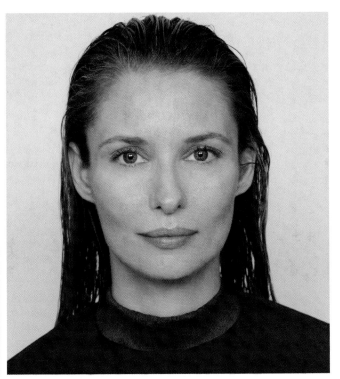

1 Start with hair that has been shampooed and conditioned. Then, apply a styling product to towel-dried hair best suited for the client's hair type and texture.

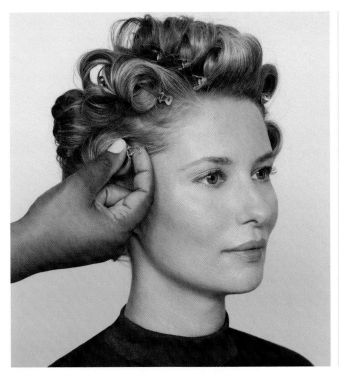

2 Blowdry the hair with a round brush. Then curl the hair with a medium-sized curling iron and clip each piece.

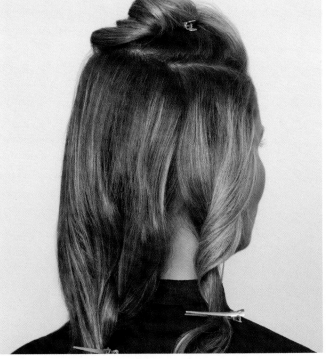

3 Divide the front hair from the back, behind the apex and ears. Then, separate the hair at the temples for the top section; the remaining hair will be the back and side sections.

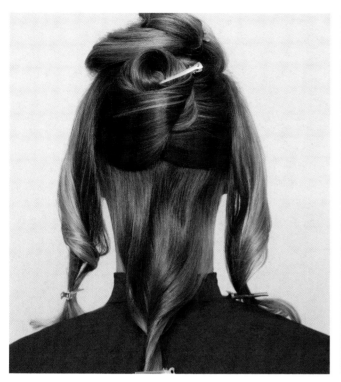

4 Subdivide the back section horizontally to just below the occipital bone.

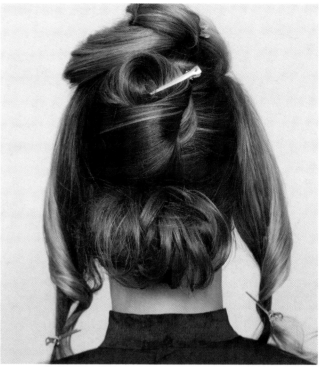

5 Tease the loose hair slightly. Divide the back subsection into 3 to 4 pieces. Each piece will be looped upward and bobby pinned. Some of the ends can be left out.

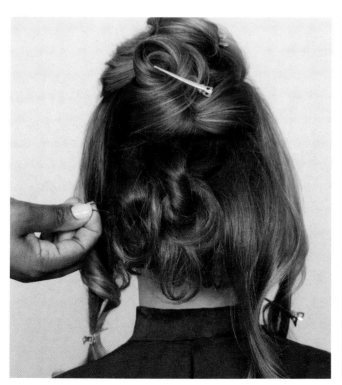

6 Subdivide the back section again and divide the hair in 3 to 4 pieces. Loop downward and pin. The partings and loops *should not* be perfect.

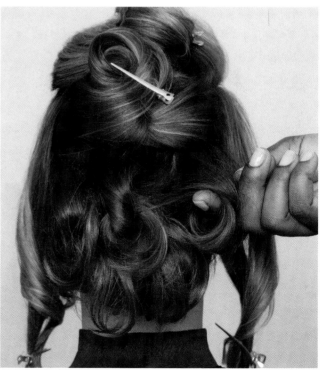

7 Loop and bobby pin the rest of the back section.

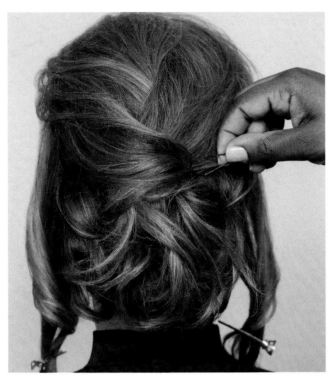

8 Tease the top section slightly. Now, take large random pieces and bobby pin into the back section until the top area is completed.

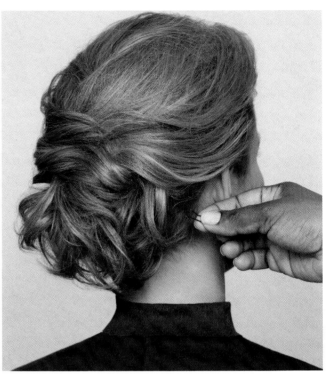

9 The sides should also be randomly pinned to the back section. Some pieces can be twisted and then pinned.

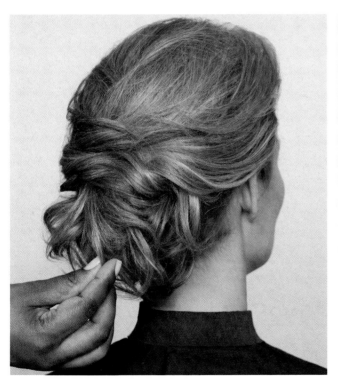

10 Make sure there are no holes visible and arrange the ends that stick out.

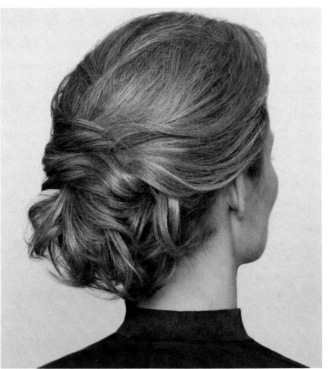

11 Finish with hair spray.

FALLEN
PIECES

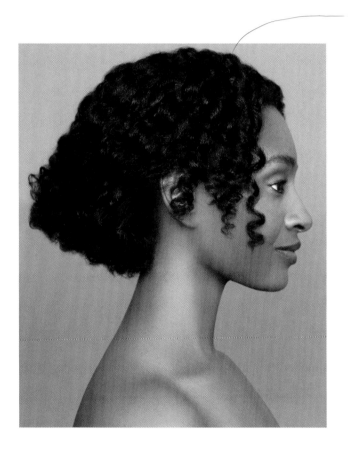
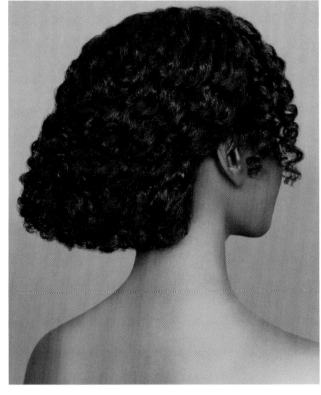

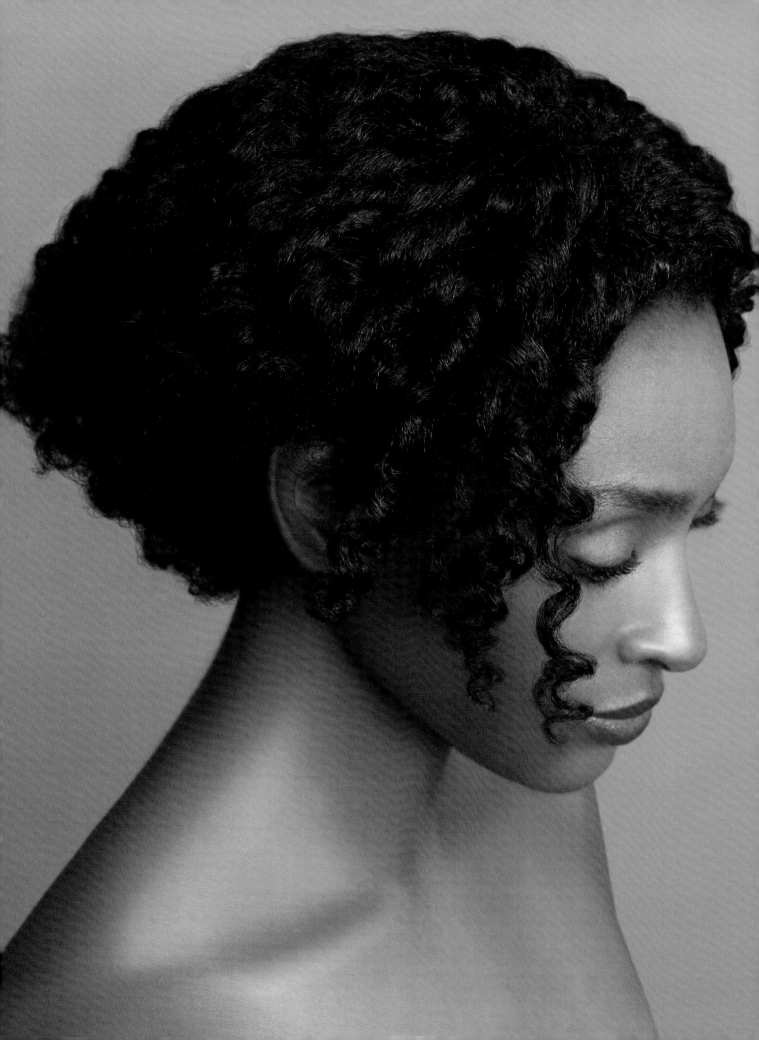

FALLEN **PIECES**

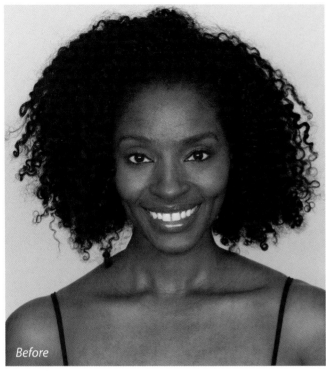

Before

Hair Texture: Curly
Hair Length: Shoulder-length

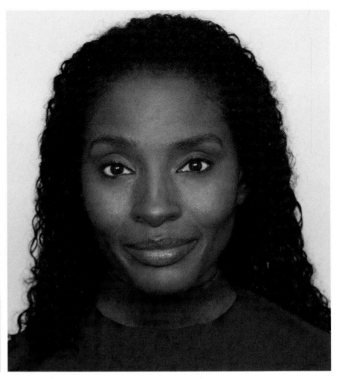

1 Start with hair that has been shampooed and conditioned. Then, apply a styling product to towel-dried hair best suited for the client's hair type and texture.

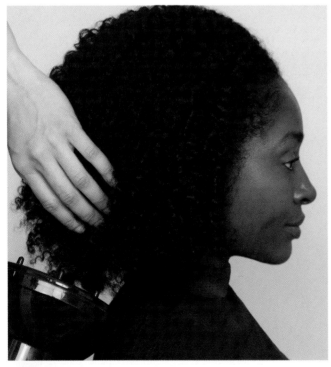

2 Dry the hair with a diffuser.

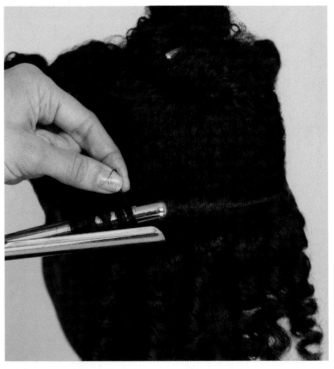

3 Curl the hair by wrapping 1-inch sections around a small curling iron.

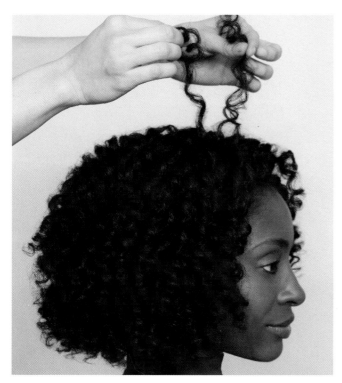

4 Separate the curls by pulling them apart.

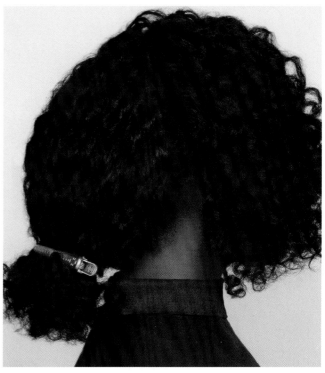

5 Divide the front hair from the back, behind the apex and ears. Establish a side parting.

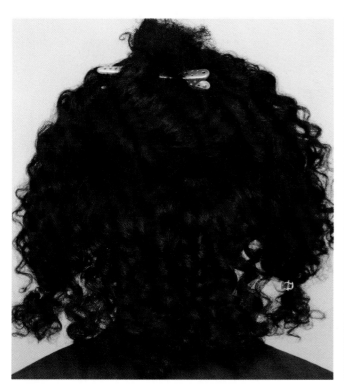

6 Divide the back section horizontally about 3 inches above the hairline.

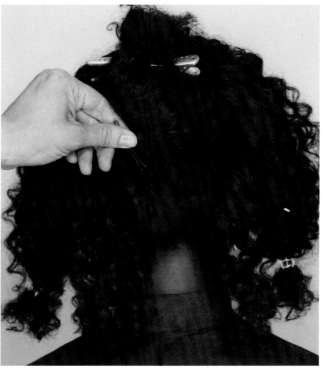

7 Subdivide the hair into 3 sections. Then, loop the middle section upward and secure with bobby pins.

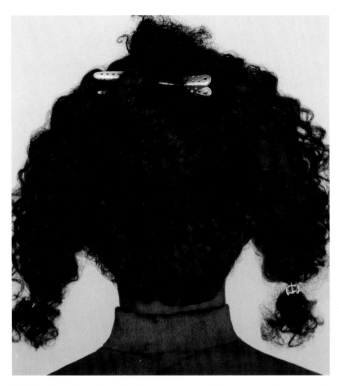

8 Loop the other 2 back sections toward the center and secure with bobby pins.

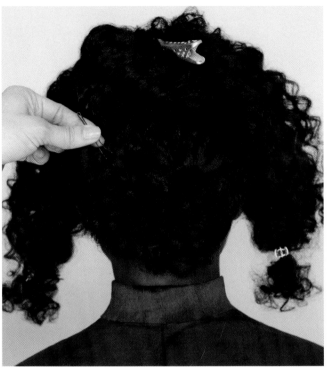

9 Divide the back section horizontally 2 inches above the previous section. Then, subdivide the hair into 2 or 3 sections and loop toward the previous looped sections. Secure with bobby pins.

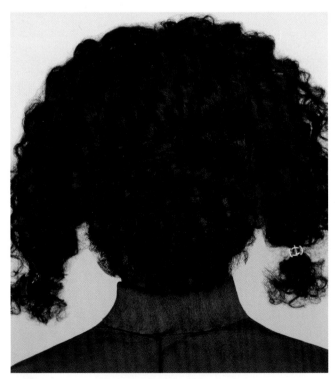

10 Finish the back section by subdividing the remaining hair into 2 sections. Loop and secure with bobby pins.

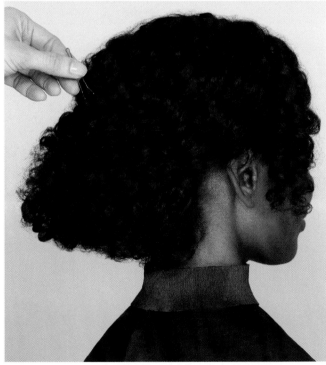

11 Subdivide the sides into 2 sections and loosely pin to the back with bobby pins. Leave hair around the face for softness.

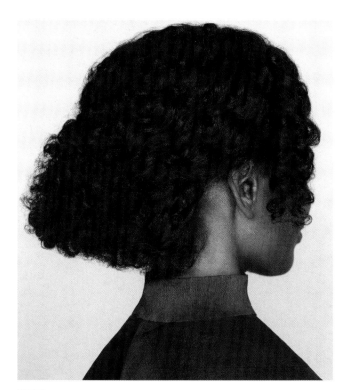

12 Finish with texture spray.

CURLY
PIECES

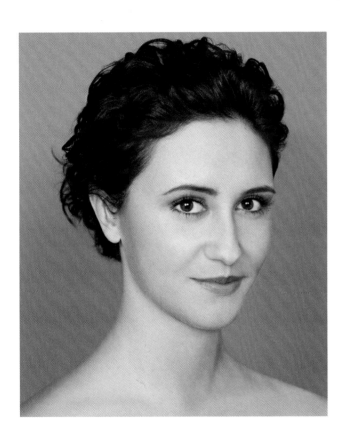
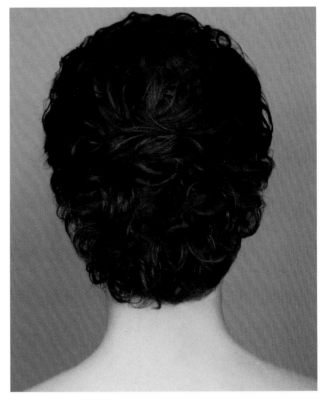

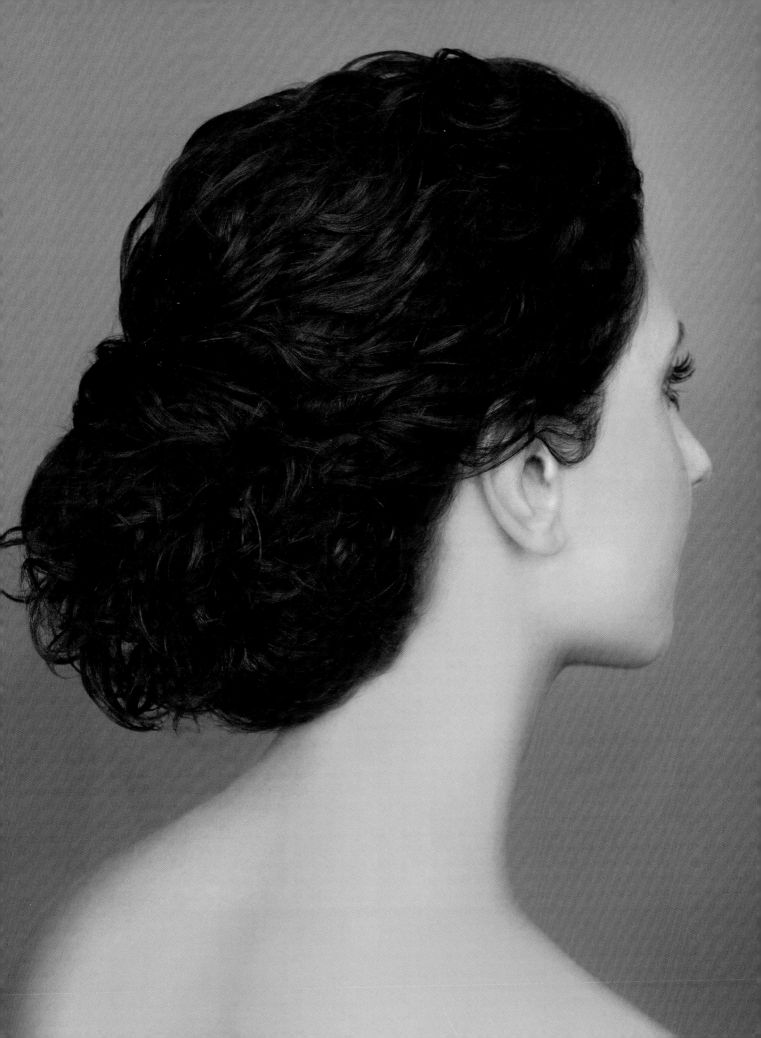

CURLY **PIECES**

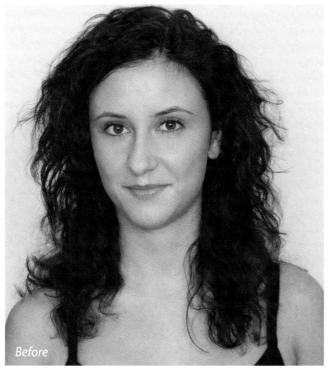

Before

Hair Texture: Curly
Hair Length: Shoulder-length

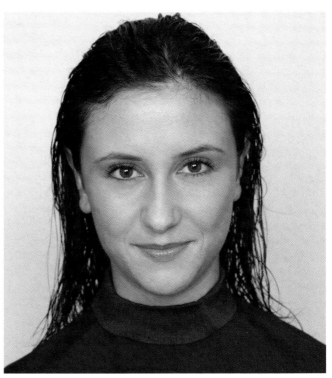

1 Start with hair that has been shampooed and conditioned. Then, apply a styling product to towel-dried hair best suited for the client's hair type and texture.

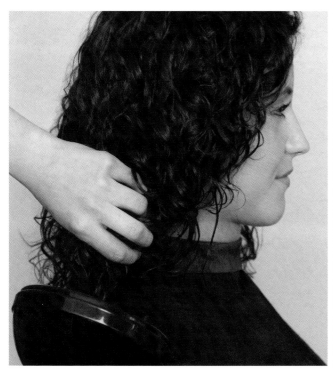

2 Dry naturally curly hair with a diffuser.

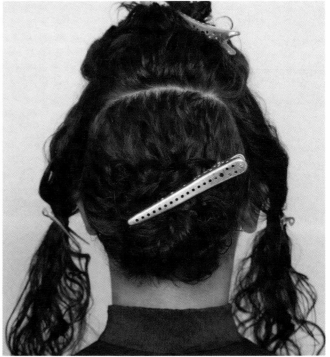

3 Divide the front hair from the back, behind the apex and ears. Then, separate the hair at the temples for the top section; the remaining hair will be the back and side sections.

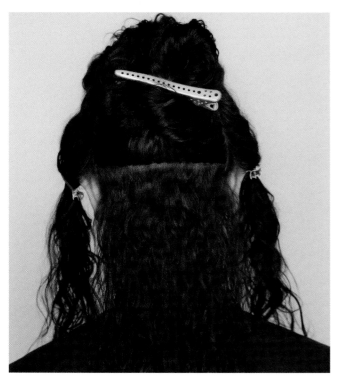

4 Subdivide the back section horizontally about 3 inches above the hairline.

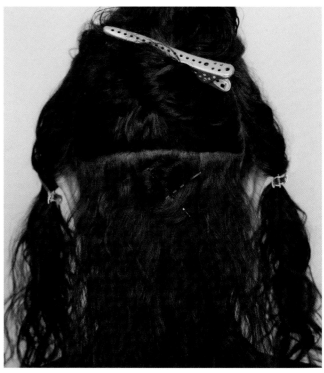

5 Take a 2-inch piece of hair from the center and make a flat pin curl. Secure it by crisscrossing two bobby pins.

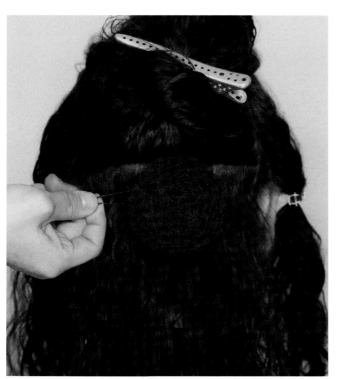

6 Attach a small filler on top of the crisscrossed pins and secure with bobby pins.

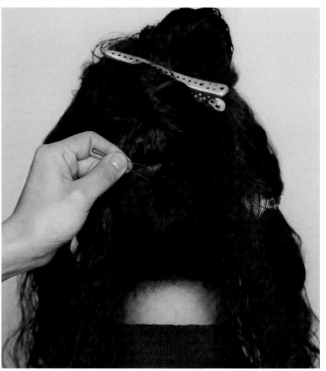

7 Starting with the center back piece, tease the hair slightly and take random pieces of hair to cover the filler.

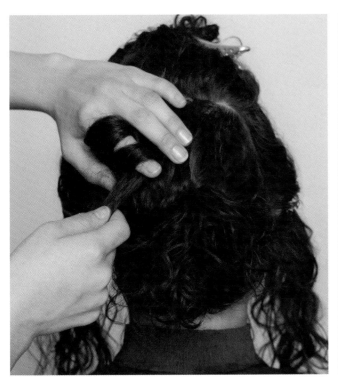

8 Finish the back section by looping and intertwining large random pieces and securing with bobby pins. Leave some of the ends out.

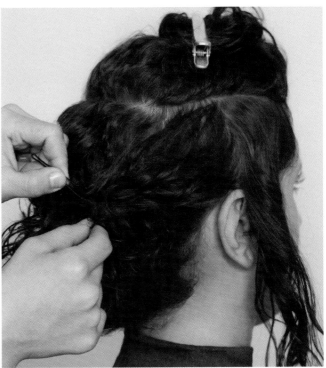

9 Subdivide the side sections into 2 pieces. Gently twist each piece and intertwine with the back section; secure with bobby pins.

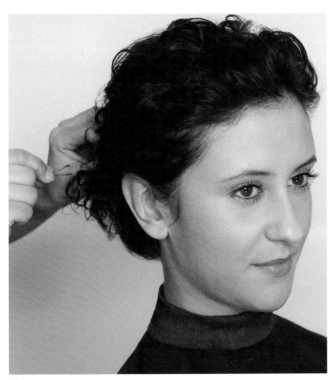

10 The top section is directed back in large random pieces and secured with bobby pins.

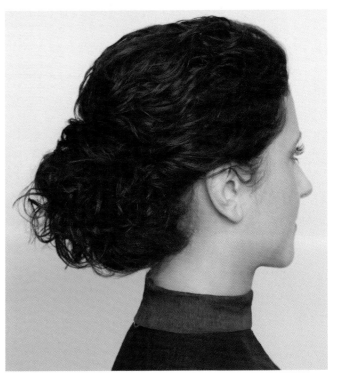

11 Finish with texture spray.

TOUSLED UP

Back in the 1950s and 1960s when nearly everyone's hair was perfectly in place, French actress Brigitte Bardot had sexy tousled hair. In all of her movies, her hairstyles were "done but undone." Bardot's hairstyles still resonate today, influencing everyone from Madonna to Beyoncé.

For this section, we chose the hairstyles Tousled Pieces, Piled Up, and Bardot. Fillers were used on all three of the hairstyles for added volume. Wefts were attached in Bardot to thicken the hair. One helpful hint is to use your hands for these tousled hairstyles because they help separate the hair.

TOUSLED
PIECES

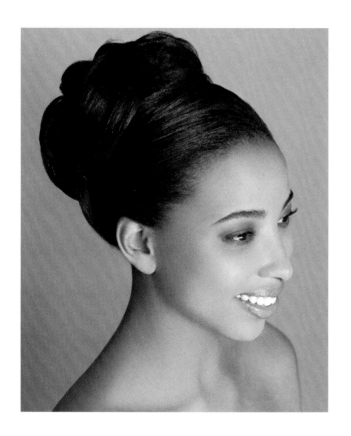
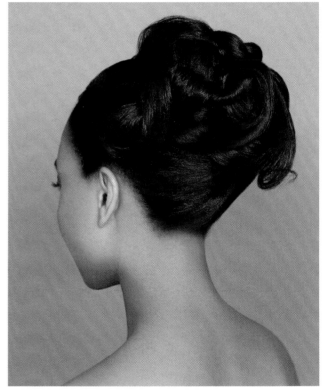

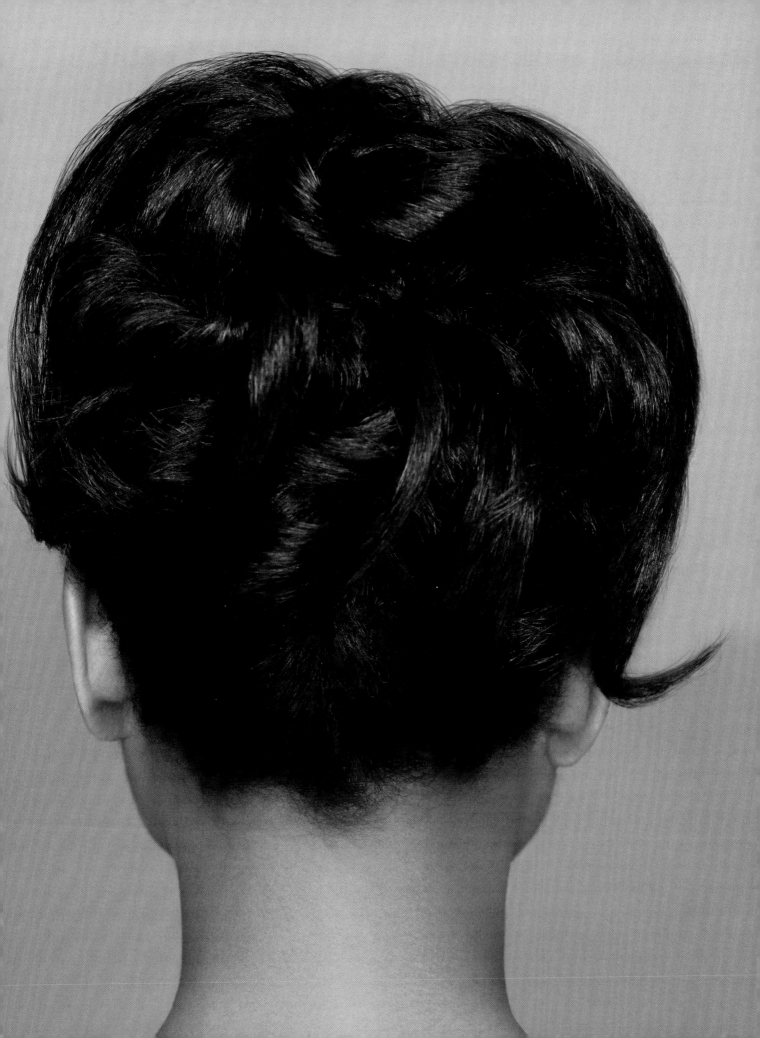

TOUSLED **PIECES**

Before

Hair Texture: Fine, straight
Hair Length: Above the shoulders

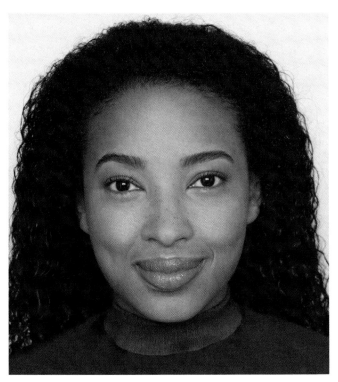

1 Start with hair that has been shampooed and conditioned. Then, apply a styling product to towel-dried hair best suited for the client's hair type and texture.

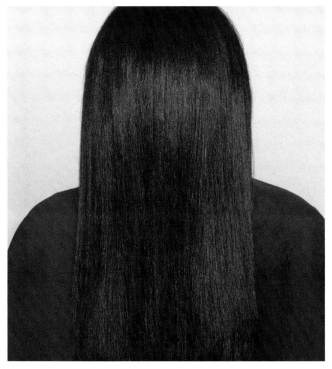

2 Blowdry the hair straight with body using a round brush.

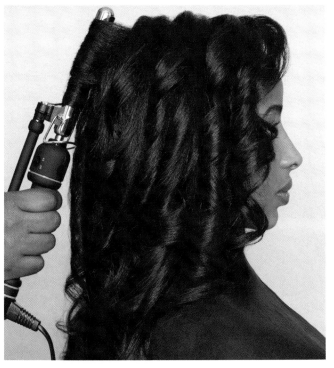

3 Curl the hair with a medium-sized curling iron.

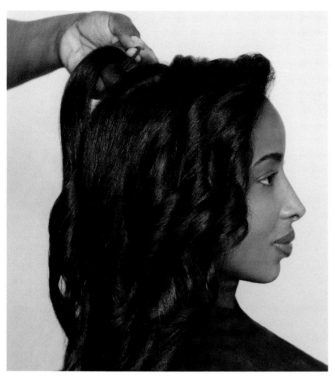

4 Make a round section on top of the head about 2 inches in diameter. It does not have to be perfect. Then, position a ponytail just below the apex.

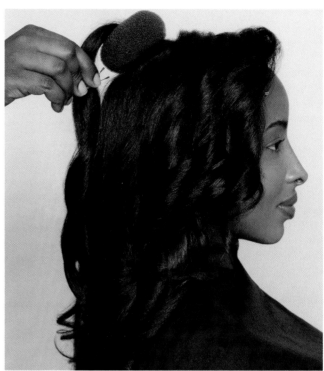

5 Pull the ponytail through a doughnut-shaped filler and secure with bobby pins.

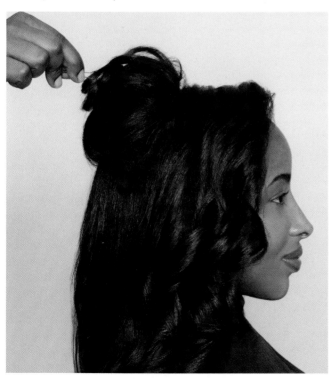

6 Tease random pieces of hair, smooth the pieces, and use them to cover the filler, securing with bobby pins.

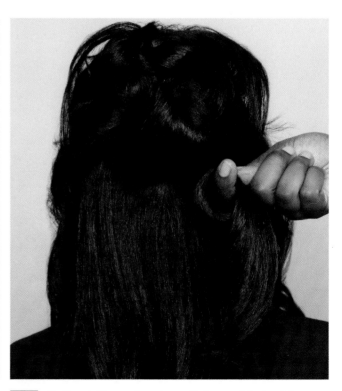

7 Continue taking random pieces of hair around the head. Loop the pieces and bobby pin them to the filler, leaving some of the ends out.

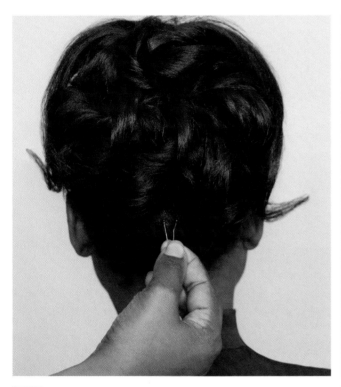

8 Tighten the nape area by twisting slightly and securing with bobby pins.

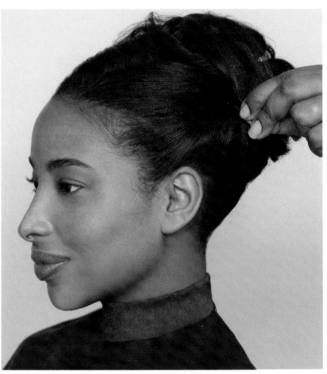

9 Tighten the sides by twisting slightly and securing with bobby pins.

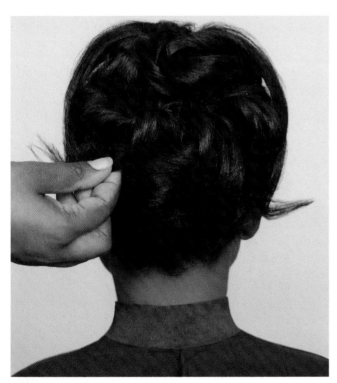

10 Arrange the loose pieces.

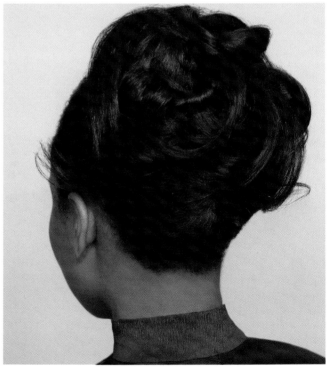

11 Finish with hair spray.

PILED
UP

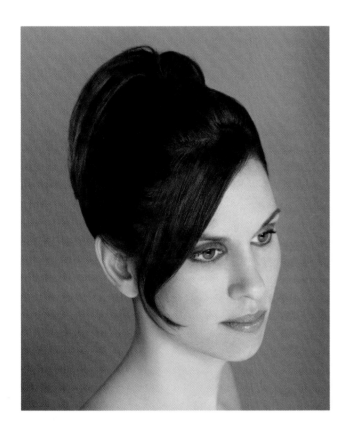
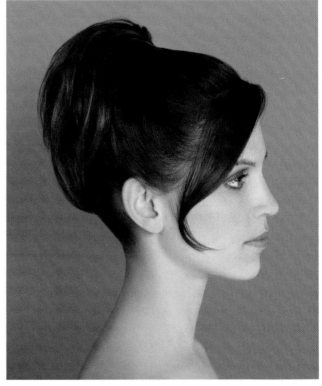

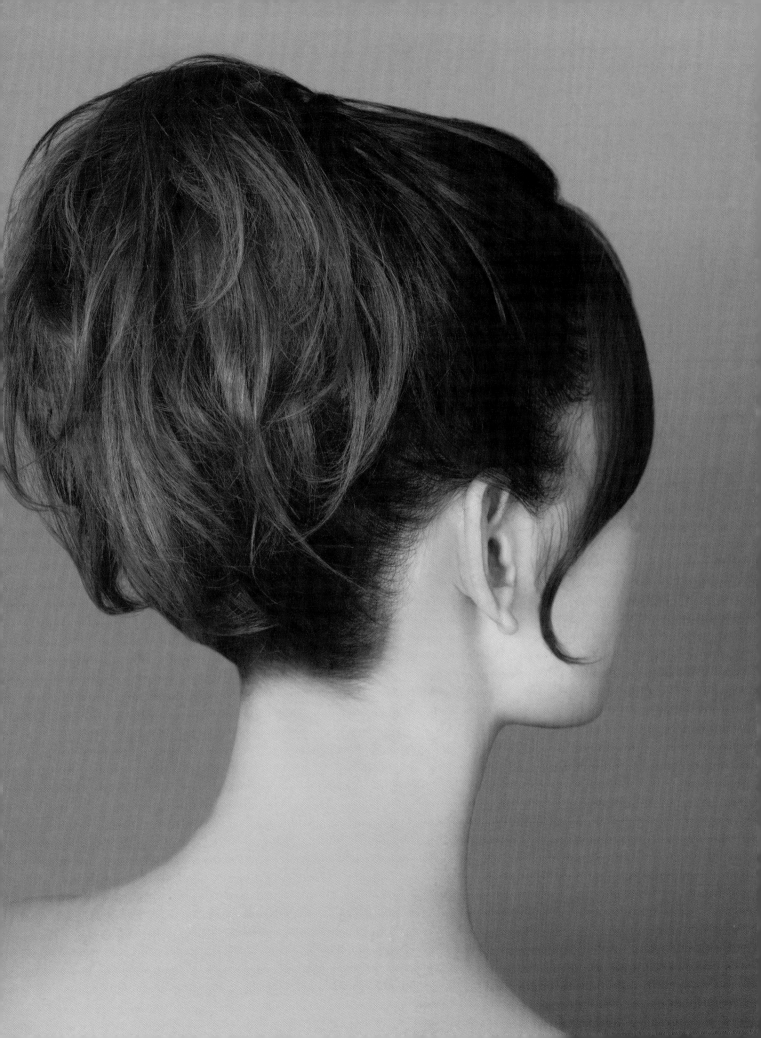

PILED **UP**

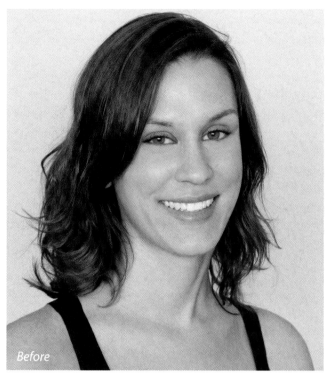

Before

Hair Texture: Thick, curly
Hair Length: Long

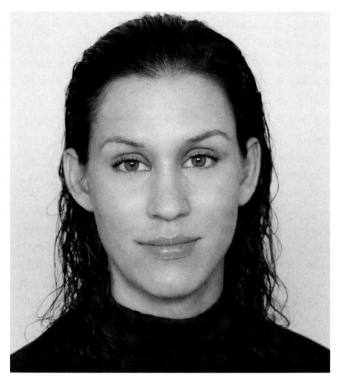

1 Start with hair that has been shampooed and conditioned. Then, apply a styling product to towel-dried hair best suited for the client's hair type and texture.

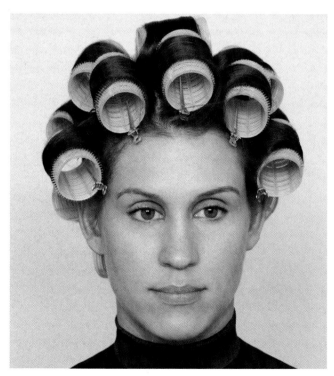

2 Blowdry the hair with a medium-sized round brush, and add Velcro rollers while drying the hair for maximum fullness.

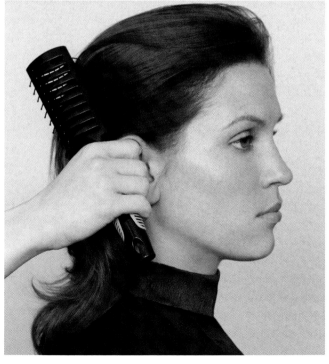

3 Remove the rollers and brush the hair thoroughly with a vent brush to remove all the parts.

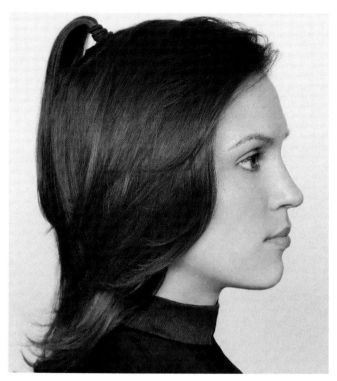

4 Make a circular section just above the apex and above the occipital. Then, make a ponytail in the center.

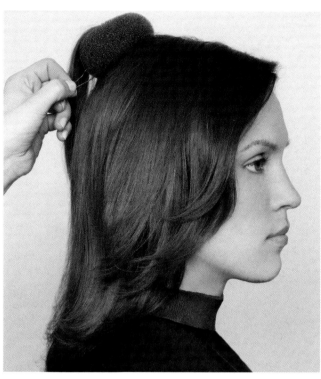

5 Pull the ponytail through a doughnut-shaped filler and secure with bobby pins.

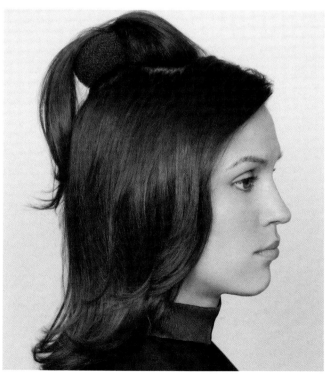

6 Starting in the front, tease a 2-inch piece of hair, twist the hair slightly, and pin it on top of the filler, leaving the ends out.

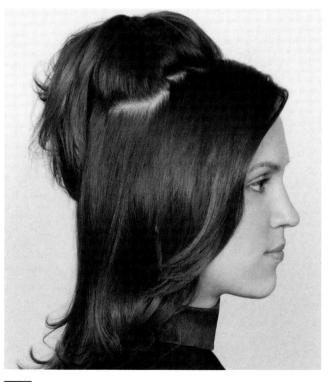

7 Work around the filler first to make sure it is concealed. Tease, twist slightly, and pin each piece on top of the filler, leaving the ends out. Some of the pieces can vary in size.

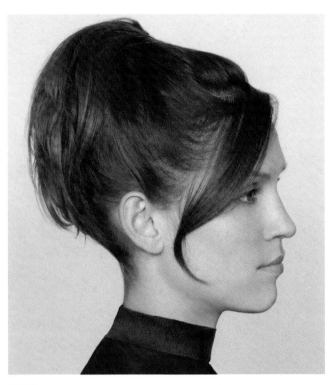

8 Keep working around the head until all the pieces are up. Leave a piece around the face for softness.

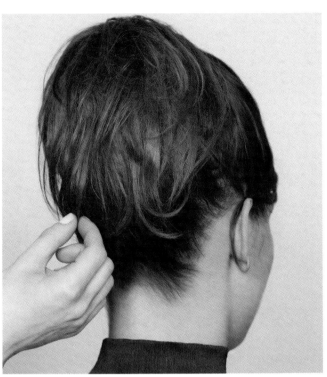

9 Arrange the ends.

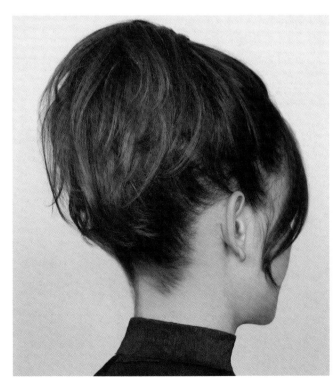

10 Finish with texture spray.

BARDOT

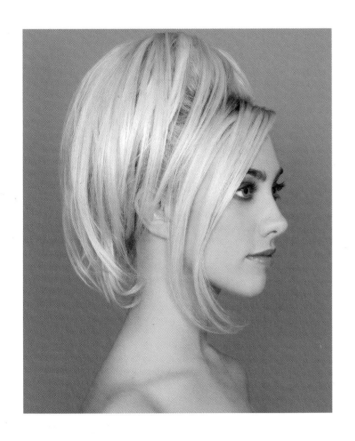
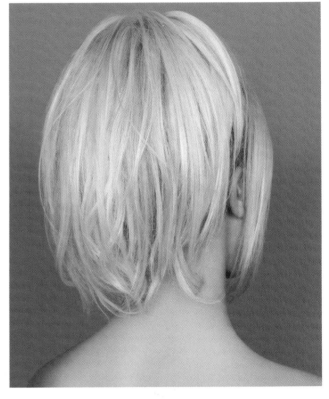

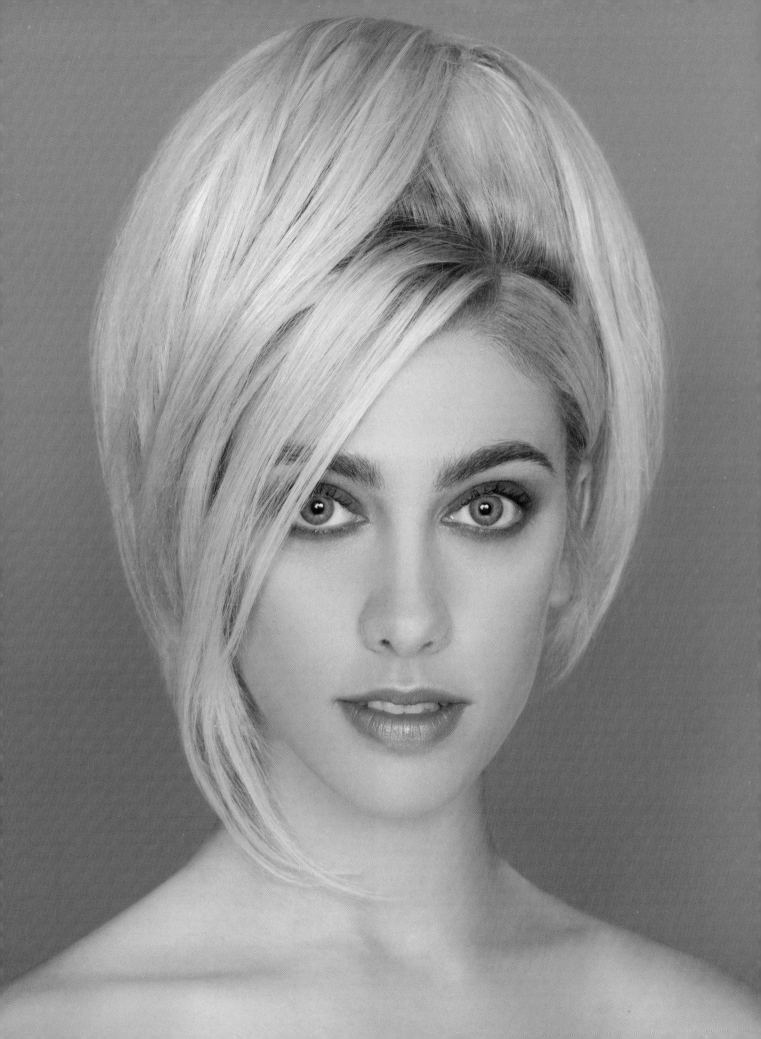

BARDOT

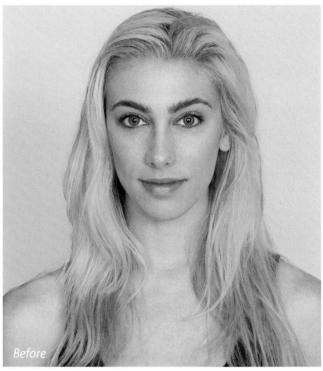

Before

Hair Texture: Fine, straight
Hair Length: Long

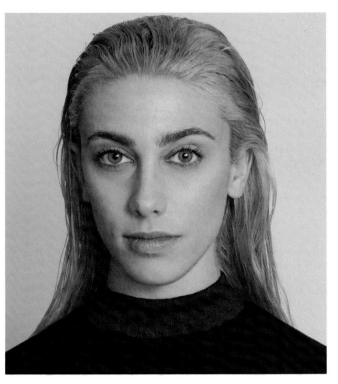

1 Start with hair that has been shampooed and conditioned. Then, apply a styling product to towel-dried hair best suited for the client's hair type and texture.

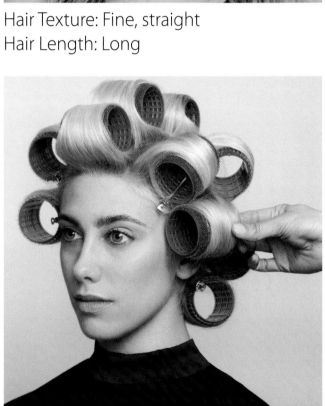

2 Blowdry the hair with a medium-sized round brush, and add Velcro rollers while drying the hair for maximum fullness.

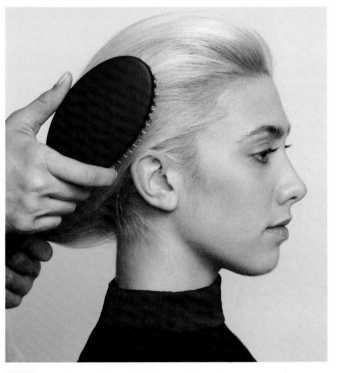

3 Remove the rollers and brush the hair thoroughly to remove all the parts.

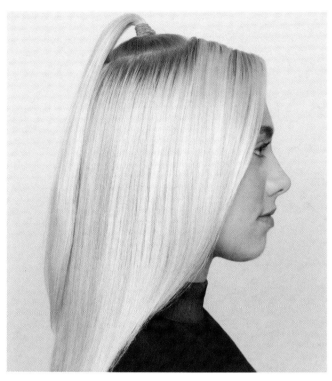

4 Make a round section on top of the head about 2 inches in diameter. It does not have to be perfect. Then, position a ponytail just in front of the apex.

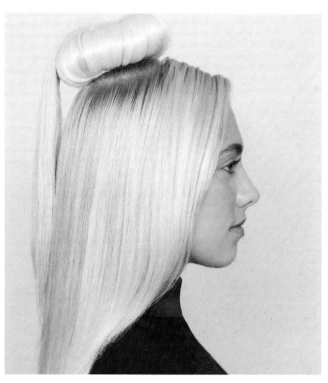

5 Pull the ponytail through a doughnut-shaped filler that has been covered with a weft that matches the client's hair color. Secure with bobby pins.

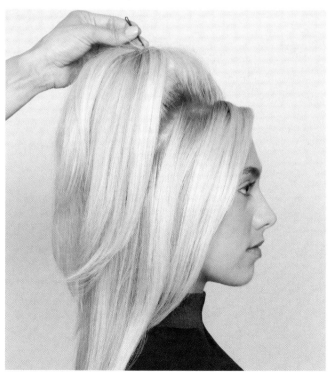

6 Tease random pieces of the client's hair and pin on top of the filler, leaving the ends loose. Work around the head.

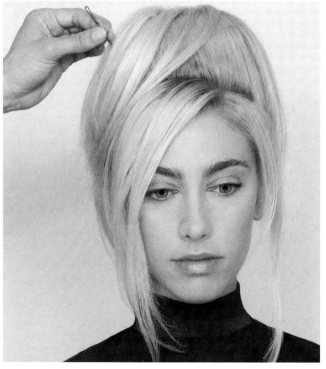

7 Finish the entire head and leave some hair around the face.

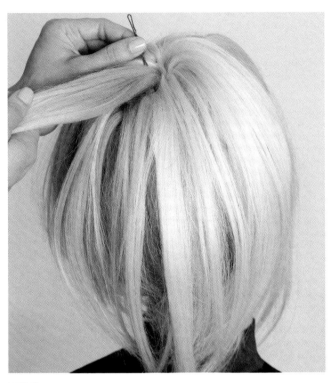

8 Add more wefts of hair around the inside of the filler and secure with bobby pins.

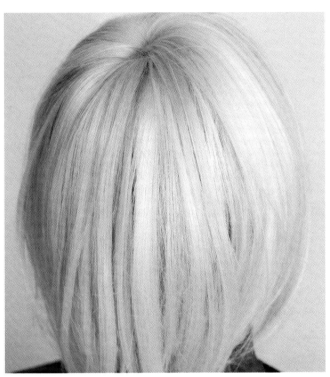

9 Distribute the ponytail on top of the wefts of hair and arrange the hair.

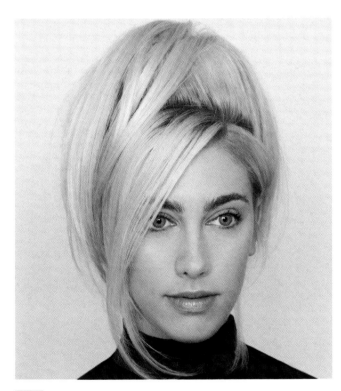

10 Finish with texture spray.